LIVING WELL WITH

Parkinson's Disease

LIVING WELL WITH

PARKINSON'S DISEASE

What Your Doctor

Doesn't Tell You . . .

That You Need to Know

**By GRETCHEN GARIE AND MICHAEL J. CHURCH
with Winifred Conkling**

A Lynn Sonberg Book

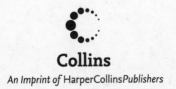

Collins
An Imprint of HarperCollins*Publishers*

HarperCollins books may be purchased for educational, business, or sales
promotional use. For information, please write: Special Markets Department, HarperCollins Publishers, 10 East 53rd Street, New York, NY
10022.

FIRST EDITION

Designed by Joy O'Meara

Library of Congress Cataloging-in-Publication Data
Garie, Gretchen.
        Living well with Parkinson's disease: what your doctor doesn't tell
you—that you need to know / by Gretchen Garie and Michael J. Church;
with Winifred Conkling. — 1st ed.
        p. cm.
        "A Lynn Sonberg Book."
        Includes bibliographical references and index.
        ISBN 978-006-117322-6
1. Parkinson's diesease—Popular works. I. Church, Michael J. II. Conkling, Winifred. III. Title.

RC382.G373 2007
616.8'33—dc22

                                        2007031034

07 08 09 10 11   ID/RRD   10 9 8 7 6 5 4 3 2 1

We would like to dedicate this book to:

Our Parents—Garrie and Mellany; Larry and Carol
Throughout our lives, you have loved us, stood by us,
and continued to support us and be our biggest cheerleaders.

**Our Siblings—Carol and Carrie;
Wendy, Rick and Annemarie**
Thank you for taking the time to understand Parkinson's disease,
for advocating on our behalf, and for being there when we needed
extra support.

**Our Children—LuLaura, Christine,
Michelle, Rebekah, and Michael, Jr.**
We hope that we have taught you that life is 10 percent what
happens to you and 90 percent how you deal with it.

Our Parkinson's Family
To those who opened their hearts and lives to share with
others in this book, we thank you. To those who have come before
us and who we hope will benefit from where we have been,
we are honored that you are a part of our lives.

MEDICAL DISCLAIMER

This book is designed to give information on Parkinson's-related conditions, treatments, and procedures for your personal knowledge and to help you be a more informed consumer of medical and health services. It is not intended to be complete or exhaustive, nor is it a substitute for the advice of your physician. You should seek medical care promptly for any specific medical condition or problem you may have. Under no circumstances should medication of any kind be administered without first checking with your physician.

All efforts have been made to ensure the accuracy of the information contained in this book as of the date published. The authors and the publisher expressly disclaim responsibility for any adverse effects arising from the use or application of the information contained herein.

The names and identifying characteristics of individuals featured throughout this book have been changed to protect their privacy.

CONTENTS

FOREWORD

By John D. Campbell, M.D.

Gretchen Garie and Michael J. Church have been my patients for more than five years. During that time, I have grown to respect their personal dedication as cofounders of the advocacy group Movers & Shakers, as well as their commitment to thriving in spite of their disease. They both willingly share their experience and expertise with those who are newly diagnosed, and they inspire all of those in the Parkinson's community to approach their lives with passion and perseverance.

In *Living Well with Parkinson's Disease*, Gretchen and Michael do an excellent job of describing both the physical and psychological changes that occur in a person with Parkinson's disease. Their firsthand knowledge as patients, coupled with their years of experience as experts and advocates, allows them to offer a unique perspective on the disease. Using the information provided by Gretchen and Michael in this book, you, too, can live well with Parkinson's disease.

Parkinson's disease is a difficult condition to live with, and one that requires a personalized approach to treatment. When I diagnose patients with Parkinson's disease, I know that they are taking the first steps of what will be a lifelong journey of acceptance and adjustment. The symptoms of Parkinson's disease—a progressive and degenerative disease caused by the loss of dopamine-producing cells in the brain—can be controlled with medication or surgery in most cases, but at present, there is no cure.

As a neurologist with a primary focus on the diagnosis and treatment of Parkinson's disease, I am witnessing the development of many new medications and procedures—some already available and others in development or clinical trial. The future looks optimistic for the treatment of Parkinson's disease patients, despite the need for a continuing search for the cause and cure of the disease. Empowered patients such as Gretchen and Michael will add strength to this search.

JOHN D. CAMPBELL, M.D., earned his medical degree at University of Saskatchewan in Canada. He did his fellowship at Cleveland Clinic in Cleveland, Ohio. He is certified by the American Board of Psychiatry and Neurology and a member of the American Academy of Neurology and the National Parkinson's Foundation.

INTRODUCTION

I was diagnosed with young-onset Parkinson's disease (YOPD) when I was 33 years old. At the time, I was living in a rural town in Tennessee, working as an autism specialist, mothering my very active preteen daughter, and trying desperately to understand why I was tired all the time and my body felt like a quivering mold of Jell-O. When the doctor finally diagnosed my condition, I felt relieved that what I was feeling had a name—but I was devastated with the reality that I faced a progressive, degenerative disease that had no cure. I had been given a life sentence with no parole.

Living in a small town with an illness such as Parkinson's was like being dropped into an Amazon tribe with no interpreter. I had no support system in my community, and my doctors were an hour away. I knew a little about Parkinson's disease (PD) because I liked Michael J. Fox, and I had read about his battle with this illness. My only other link to knowledge about PD came through the computer.

Sometimes well-intentioned friends would ask, "Are you getting better?"

I wanted to scream, "No! I'm not getting better—and I never will!" Few of the people I knew understood the disease or how to be supportive of someone with a chronic illness. There were good days, when I felt almost like my old self—and there were hopeless days, when I keenly felt the loss of my former life. Most of all, I felt alone.

I was so afraid of not being able to do things with my daughter, of gradually withering away into less than I used to be. I had to remake myself and discover new sources of spiritual strength, but these things didn't happen for me overnight.

About two years into my illness, I was approached by Michael J. Church, from Naples, Florida, who had seen some of my online postings on various Parkinson's message boards. Michael was a single father of four who had been diagnosed with Parkinson's disease when he was 32 years old. He asked me if I would assist him in starting an online support group for young people with PD. We started an online group on AOL and within three months we had more than 100 members. About a year later, we decided to expand the support we were offering from the computer monitor to the living rooms of many other people. That concept evolved, and in December 2002 Movers & Shakers was born.

The mission of Movers & Shakers is simple: to support and advocate for people with young-onset Parkinson's disease. To that end, we recruit advocates from all over the country to raise awareness about Parkinson's within their states, cities, and communities, to assist people with PD in getting the treatment they need, and to help medical professionals and others learn how to work in cooperation with those of us diagnosed with this disease. We offer online support groups, patient assistance, state advocacy programs, medical equipment exchanges, assistance with local support group start-ups, and conferences. We want to empower others to see that there is life with Parkinson's disease; we want our lives to be testimony to the reality that people with Parkinson's can live vibrant, powerful, meaningful lives. Parkinson's does not define who we are or how we live; our hands may tremble and we may stumble and fall—literally—but we are stronger than this disease.

This book, *Living Well with Parkinson's Disease*, is one that Michael and I wish we could have read when we were first diagnosed. It is a comprehensive guide that provides detailed information about the medical, emotional, financial, and practical aspects of

Parkinson's disease, both young-onset and the traditional form of the illness. The experience of living with PD is very different when you're diagnosed at age 34 than when you are diagnosed at age 64. This book strives to address and respect the challenges faced by people with this illness regardless of age.

Part 1 provides information about what Parkinson's disease is, who gets it, and how it is diagnosed. Unlike other books, this one presents the information through the prism of personal experience, as well as including anecdotes and reflections from dozens of people who are living well with PD.

Part 2 offers an overview of traditional medical care, including medication, surgery, and how to find a good doctor. Parkinson's disease can be quirky and difficult to manage; input from other people with Parkinson's can help you take advantage of the collective wisdom of those who understand the challenges you face when adjusting your medications, contemplating surgery, and finding a doctor who truly understands your condition.

Part 3 covers alternative medicine and self-care, from exercise and diet to supplements and mind-body therapies. It also includes a discussion of depression and the importance of support groups. Far too often those of us with Parkinson's disease feel alone and isolated; our hope is that this book can help you feel part of a broader community of people who truly understand your daily struggles.

In our opinion, Part 4, "Surviving and Thriving with Parkinson's Disease," sets this book apart from others on the shelf. In this section, you will receive useful information about how to *live* with Parkinson's disease. It is both pragmatic and personal. We offer practical suggestions on how to handle everyday challenges such as cutting meat or rolling over in bed, as well as ways that Parkinson's disease will change almost every personal relationship you have. We provide tips on facing job loss and maneuvering the bureaucratic maze of the Social Security Administration, as well as ways you will have to discover yourself anew as a person with Parkinson's disease.

It is our sincere hope that this book will help you live well and thrive as a person with Parkinson's disease. Parkinson's has forced us to redefine who we are and what we want out of life. While we would eliminate Parkinson's disease from our lives—and yours—if we could, in many ways we must acknowledge that the wretched disease has made us stronger. We have learned to stand up for ourselves, to take care of ourselves, and to laugh at ourselves more than we ever did before we had PD. We have learned to speak out, stand out, and act out, when necessary. We may not always be able to stop our hands from trembling, but we can lend a hand to someone who needs help.

Both Michael and I have often said: "I have Parkinson's disease, but it doesn't have me." We hope that this book will help you better understand the unique challenges you must face as a person with Parkinson's, and, more important, that it will help you imagine new possibilities of who you can be as you rediscover yourself. Like us, you have PD—but it doesn't have you.

Note: Michael and I are partners in most things that we do. He is the executive director of Movers & Shakers; I am the president. In the years that we have worked together, we have also become a family. We are on a journey together, both as advocates for people with Parkinson's disease and as life partners dedicated to helping each other overcome life's obstacles.

Many sections of this book are written in the first person, from my (Gretchen's) point of view. Michael owns these words as much as I do, but for the sake of clarity, the text reads as if it is from the perspective of a single author.

LIVING WELL WITH

Parkinson's Disease

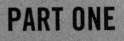

PART ONE

Diagnosis

1

What Is Parkinson's Disease?

For me, Parkinson's disease started with a twitch in the pinkie of my right hand. I stared down at my finger, willing it to behave but unable to stop the incessant flutter. I was 32 years old, and I never considered that I might have Parkinson's disease.

I did suspect that something was wrong with me. For months I had tired easily. My legs hurt during the day and felt restless at night. I felt like I was shaking on the inside and there was nothing I could do to make it stop. I went from one doctor to another, enduring tests for Lyme disease, lupus, Wilson's Disease, and sleep apnea. The results were all negative. Some people told me it was all in my head; I started to believe them. When your whole world feels crazy, it's easy to question your sanity.

Finally, a doctor wrote me a prescription for Sinemet, a drug used to treat Parkinson's patients. Within days, my fingers stilled, my insides quieted, and I felt like myself again. My doctor then told me two things: I definitely had Parkinson's disease—and I could not use the drug that gave me that brief period of physical relief. He explained that this was a strong medication but that it has side effects that appear after several years' use; I should use other, somewhat less effective medications for as long as possible, saving the stronger drugs for when I needed them most. I felt the double blow of a cruel diagnosis and a cruel treatment regimen.

Michael's diagnosis came as very unwelcome news on his 32nd birthday. For several years, his legs had shaken and wobbled uncontrollably during periods of stress or conflict. He tried to minimize stress by quitting his job as director of an insurance school in Florida and switching to a retail management position. "Sales quotas and other high-stress expectations seemed to trigger the same weak-in-the-knees symptoms, which I ignored again," he said. "A year and a half passed, and the symptoms grew progressively more frequent and more intense." He also noticed a twitch of the two smallest fingers of his left hand. The more intense the stress, the more intense his symptoms became.

Michael saw a morning television program that mentioned a thyroid disorder causing similar symptoms. His doctor performed various tests, all of which were inconclusive. He was referred to a neurologist, who prescribed a three-day course of Sinemet. At the follow-up appointment, he told his doctor he felt much better—and the doctor told him he had young-onset Parkinson's disease.

"I remember thinking, 'Is this right? Isn't that a senior's disease? There must be some mistake,'" said Michael. "This was an unwanted birthday present, and it began what I consider to be the biggest challenge of my life."

In the years since then, Michael and I have had to become experts on living with Parkinson's disease. We have learned a great deal about what it is and how it affects the body. This chapter will cover the basics of PD and how it affects the brain, muscles, and neurological system.

▮ Dopamine and the Brain

In the simplest terms, Parkinson's disease is a movement disorder in which the brain doesn't have enough of the chemical dopamine to help transmit nerve impulses throughout the body. It is a degenerative condition; you'll have good days and bad days, but over the years, your condition will worsen as more and more dopamine-producing cells are destroyed.

In your day-to-day life, Parkinson's will present a number of physical challenges, depending on which symptoms you have. The three classic motor symptoms of Parkinson's disease are tremor (shaking), rigidity (stiffness), and bradykinesia (slowness). (The symptoms of Parkinson's disease are described in detail in Chapter 3.)

Doctors often claim that the symptoms of Parkinson's don't hurt, but I know for a fact that isn't true. On many days, my muscles and joints ache. Karen M., 56, agrees: "Parkinson's does hurt. Doctors may tell you it doesn't hurt, but they don't live with it so they don't really know. I haven't been comfortable for at least five years. My muscles tighten and become stiff. Sometimes it's very painful and other times it's just uncomfortable."

For most people with Parkinson's disease, their symptoms will come and go, hour by hour, day by day. "People see you when your medication is 'on' and you're walking around and looking almost normal, and so they think you're faking it when you're 'off,'" said Karen. "My daughter said to me, 'You can get up and get going when you want to go to the flea market, but not when we need to go where I want to go.' Unfortunately, it's hard for other people to understand that things can change from minute to minute."

When symptoms are active, Parkinson's disease can make it difficult to button a shirt, rise from a chair, roll over in bed, walk to the bathroom, or sign a letter. When symptoms are inactive or under control with medication, it may be impossible to detect that someone has Parkinson's disease.

Typically, the disease progresses slowly, taking several years before symptoms become significant enough to cause serious disability. However, Parkinson's disease will change your life from the moment of diagnosis. While the initial physical symptoms may be mild, the psychological challenges are often toughest to deal with early in the disease. Medication may hide the outward symptoms of Parkinson's disease for many years, but a person may be suffering emotionally during this time. Most people wrestle with feelings of betrayal ("How can my body do this to me?"), injustice ("Why me?"), anger ("It's not fair!"), and fear ("What will become of me? How will I survive?").

Marian, 60, has found it difficult to make other people understand how her condition can change throughout the day. "My friends and family expect me to be the same person I was before, but I'm not the same mentally or physically," she said. "When my medication controls my tremors and outward symptoms, I look like the same person I was, but I'm not inside. I look the same, but I'm not the same person anymore."

These physical and emotional changes take place in a person with Parkinson's disease when the dopamine-producing cells in the substantia nigra compacta, a region in the middle of the brain, die off. This is the part of the brain responsible for regulation of motor activity. In a healthy adult, about 1,200 of the 400,000 dopamine-producing neurons die each year; in a person with Parkinson's disease, the rate of cell death is dramatically higher. The signs of Parkinson's disease typically appear when about 70 to 80 percent of these cells have been destroyed. As more of these cells die, the symptoms of Parkinson's disease worsen.

In order for movement to take place, messages must be passed along a series of neurological pathways; if there is a "short" along this electrical circuit, the message cannot be sent or received, thwarting smooth movement. Dopamine is a chemical in the brain that facilitates the transmission of these messages. When dopamine levels drop, message transfer slows down or stops.

In addition to the destruction of the dopamine-producing cells, other neurochemical changes occur in the brain of a person with Parkinson's disease. The parts of the brain known as the dorsal motor nucleus of the vagus and the locus ceruleus also degenerate; in addition, levels of the neurotransmitters norepinephrine and serotonin decline. These changes account for some of the other symptoms—such as depression—that often accompany Parkinson's disease. (Depression is discussed in Chapter 11.)

The primary treatments involve the use of medication to restore dopamine levels (see Chapter 4 for more information) or surgery to reprogram the brain's electrical circuitry (see Chapter 5 for more information).

▌ The Stages of Parkinson's Disease

While the physical progression of Parkinson's symptoms may be slow, the emotional changes can be overwhelming from the start. The first two years after diagnosis are critical for doing all you can to come to terms with the illness. This involves learning about the illness, comparing medications, accepting support from others who understand what you are going through, finding a good neurologist or movement-disorders specialist, and working with your family to deal with the upcoming changes.

Most people won't notice major changes in their symptoms on a day-to-day basis, but over a period of years symptoms become worse. Your tremors will become more exaggerated, your muscles may feel stiffer, or you may feel less steady on your feet. Of course, the disease is expressed differently in different people, but most people experience these changes over time. Fortunately, doctors can customize and modify the treatment program to minimize the changing symptoms.

In most cases, people with Parkinson's become disabled and unable to work in five to ten years after diagnosis, although the disease progresses more slowly in some people and much faster in others. I had rapid progression PD and was only able to work about two years after diagnosis, while Michael worked for seven years before he was unable to do his job. Parkinson's disease is highly individualized.

Typically, symptoms appear first on one side of the body, affecting the opposite side only after years or decades have passed. "The first thing I noticed was my pinkie twitching on my right hand when I was carrying my two-year-old son," said Karen M. "I thought to myself, 'This is a brain thing, not a finger thing.' Later my right arm would shake a little, and I started to drag my right foot."

At first, symptoms will probably be mild enough that they may be ignored; in fact, most people have some minor symptoms for years before they are diagnosed. Karen M. suspects she had slow progression of her PD for 10 or 12 years before she needed to consult a neurologist. "I worked in the health-care field, and I was reasonably sure of what I had. I just didn't want to hear it, so I hid it. I'm just stubborn."

Kellie suspects that her Parkinson's symptoms first appeared at age 29, three years before her diagnosis. "I couldn't keep my head still," said Kellie. "No one wanted to say anything, and I reached a point I didn't really notice it. One day my daughter, who was about four years old, grabbed my face and said, 'Mom, please stop your jerking.' At that point I knew something was wrong."

To assess the progression of the disease, doctors tend to refer to a system of staging known as the modified Hoehn and Yahr staging scale. This allows doctors to monitor the progression of the disease over time. The scale is also used to track patients involved in various clinical studies.

Before reviewing the scale, keep several things in mind. First, most people who have had Parkinson's disease for several years actually fit into several different stages, depending on the day or the medications they are taking. Even people who may be assessed at stages 4 or 5 can often be downgraded to stage 2 or 3 once they receive the appropriate medication or other treatment. In other words, it is essential that you find a good doctor who views your treatment as a dynamic process that will change over time as your symptoms and needs change. Hope and help are available, but you may need to experiment with various medications and dosages until you find the right treatment for you.

According to the scale, I would have stage 4 Parkinson's disease. I have bilateral tremors that often interfere with daily living skills, such as dressing, cooking, and other tasks. I lose my balance, and while I can walk and stand on my own, I require a cane and even a scooter at times for mobility and balance. While most days I can complete bathing, dressing, and living tasks with minimal, if any, assistance, there are people nearby in case I do need help.

The Stages of Parkinson's Disease

Stage 0	No sign of disease
Stage 1	Unilateral disease (affecting either left or right side of the body); symptoms mild
Stage 1.5	Unilateral disease and axial (neck and back/trunk)
Stage 2	Mild bilateral (left and right) disease, without impairment of balance
Stage 2.5	Mild bilateral disease, with some mild imbalance
Stage 3	Mild to moderate bilateral disease with some difficulty with balance, still physically independent
Stage 4	Moderate to severe bilateral disease with marked disability (needs help with most motor daily tasks such as dressing, bathing, eating); still able to walk or stand without a person assisting, but may need a cane or walker; unable to live alone
Stage 5	Advanced disease, wheelchair bound or bedridden; requires nursing care; may experience malnutrition

▌ Parkinson-Plus Syndromes

In rare cases, people thought to suffer from Parkinson's disease are later found to suffer from a group of neurodegenerative illnesses often referred to as Parkinson-plus syndromes or atypical Parkinson's disease. These conditions—including progressive supranuclear palsy, striatonigral degeneration, multiple systems atrophy (cerebellar and parkinsonian types), cortiobasal ganglionic degeneration, and diffuse Lewy body disease—resemble Parkinson's disease is some ways, but they are clinically distinct. For example:

▌ Symptoms usually appear on both the right and left sides.
▌ Tremor is rarely present.
▌ Symptoms tend to progress rapidly, resulting in significant disability within five years.
▌ Symptoms are resistant to most medications for Parkinson's disease.
▌ Severe loss of balance is common.
▌ Symptoms often include difficulty swallowing, speaking, and moving the eyes.

When I was first diagnosed with Parkinson's disease, my symptoms progressed rapidly. At one point, my doctor thought that I suffered from Parkinson-plus syndrome; I was told that I had less than seven years to live. My daughter was a teenager, and all I could think of was not being alive to see her graduate from college, to attend her wedding, or to hold my grandchildren some day. My depression grew worse—but over time my symptoms slowed. For reasons no one fully understands, my condition became less threatening, and my current movement-disorders specialist reversed the diagnosis. He felt that my condition was within the spectrum of Parkinson's disease, with a few autonomic system twists. This time the diagnosis came as a great relief.

▌ You Are Not Alone ▌

Experts estimate that 1 million Americans have Parkinson's disease, a condition first identified by English physician James Parkinson in 1817 and named "the shaking palsy." Unfortunately, this number is just an estimate—and probably too low—because there is no national registry for Parkinson's disease. We know that every nine minutes someone is told that they have Parkinson's disease, including 1 out of every 100 people over age 60; last year at least 60,000 were diagnosed. There is some progress toward creating a national registry. Currently there is a voluntary registry operated by the Muhammad Ali Parkinson Center, and people with Parkinson's are encouraged to register there (www.maprc.com).

Parkinson's disease affects men and women, although it is slightly more common in men. While most people think of Parkinson's disease as a condition of the elderly, the median age at the time of onset is 45—a figure that has been declining in recent years. Young-onset Parkinson's disease is defined at diagnosis before age 55—and about 15 percent of all cases of Parkinson's are early-onset. It is disturbing that the number of people being diagnosed before age 45 is growing, and this phenomenon has not been explained.

▌ What Causes Parkinson's Disease?

While researchers have lots of theories about the cause of Parkinson's disease, no one really knows for sure. Most experts theorize that the disease is not caused by a single factor, but rather by a combination of inherited risk with some kind of environmental factor, such as a virus, exposure to a toxin, or some kind of stress to the body. In other words, to develop the disease, a person would have to have both a genetic predisposition and exposure to some other environmental risk factor. This so-called double-hit hypothesis suggests that more than one condition must be met for a person to develop Parkinson's disease. Some neurologists phrase it this way: "Genetics loads the gun, and the environment pulls the trigger."

Most people with Parkinson's disease have no idea what may have caused the disease to be expressed. Some, like Karen R., believe that exposure to chemicals may have brought on the disease: "I grew up on a farm, and a local farmer rented the field around our house," she said. "He used tons of pesticides and herbicides and that was the source of our water supply."

Sarah, 59, sees several possible causes for her PD. "I grew up in southern Indiana when pesticides were all over the bread basket," she said. "I also wonder if the trigger event for me was damage done in the womb, since my mother fell when she was pregnant. My right side is smaller than my left—my left foot is larger, my breast is larger, and scans show my left brain is larger."

Most people with Parkinson's ultimately make peace with the idea that they will probably never know what constellation of events made them vulnerable to the disease. While most of us cannot help but ask ourselves the what-if questions, ultimately we must face the challenges present in our daily struggles of living with the disease. We can't change the past, but we can make the best of our futures.

The Role of Oxidative Stress

Oxidative stress is caused by free radicals, unstable molecules in the body that have the power to damage other molecules. They can injure cell proteins and DNA, and sometimes cause cell death. Many experts believe oxidative stress may play a major role in the death of dopamine-producing cells in the brain.

The immune system tries to seek out and destroy free radicals, but when the immune system is taxed or weakened, it can't keep up with the demand. Antioxidant nutrients—such as the nutritional supplements vitamin C and E—help neutralize free radicals before they cause harm.

Researchers know that in the brain dopamine is broken down into peroxides, which in turn form free radicals. Those peroxides can be detoxified by glutathione. If the level of peroxides is too high or the level of glutathione is too low, then oxidative stress and cause cell death—ultimately resulting in Parkinson's disease.

In the fall of 2006, researchers found that blocking one of the body's natural inflammatory factors helped protect against brain cell death similar to that found in PD. In laboratory studies on rats, a drug found to inhibit an inflammatory molecule known as tumor necrosis factor (TNF) resulted in a 50 percent drop in the death of dopamine-producing cells in the brain. TNF is an essential part of a healthy immune system, but it also appears to play a role in the development of PD. In fact, high levels of TNF are found in the brains and cerebrospinal fluid of people with PD after they die. In the future, the drug may be used to slow the progression of Parkinson's disease; further modifications are needed before it can be used on humans because at this time the drug cannot cross the blood-brain barrier, a protective feature that does not allow certain types of molecules to cross into the brain.

The Role of Mitochondria

In 1983, researchers began to consider the possibility that mitochondria—the energy production centers of the cells—might play a role in Parkinson's disease. That year, Parkinson-like symptoms appeared in drug users who injected an illegal drug known as MPTP. In the body, MPTP is broken down into MPP+, a toxic substance known to destroy dopamine-producing cells in the brain by altering the cells' mitochondria. If the destruction of the mitochondria caused Parkinson-like symptoms in these people, perhaps it also plays a role in actual Parkinson's disease.

What other substances interfere with the mitochondria? Researchers know that some pesticides and herbicides, carbon monoxide, hydrogen sulfide, cyanide, and nitric acid, among others, all damage the mitochondria. In addition, many of these substances have been linked to Parkinson's disease.

Excitotoxicity

Excessive stimulation of the brain by the excitatory chemical glutamate may contribute to the death of cells in the substantia nigra. Glutamate appears to excite the cell and increase the flow of calcium to the cell, which in turn activates enzymes that break down cell proteins and destroy the brain cells. (Dopamine cells have a large number of glutamate receptors.)

Animal studies involving rats and monkeys have shown that animals given drugs to block glutamate activity do not develop parkinsonian symptoms when given drugs designed to trigger cell death. In other words, blocking glutamate may protect the brain cells from toxic damage. This is an area currently under investigation.

The Presence of Lewy Body

A healthy brain does not contain Lewy bodies; the brain of someone with Parkinson's disease does. Lewy bodies are clumps of proteins that affect cell function and assist in the breakdown of larger proteins. It's not clear whether the Lewy bodies form when the cells in the brain die or if the Lewy bodies in fact contribute to the cell death in the first place.

Ubiquitin is a protein found in the Lewy body. Ubiquitin binds to old or damaged proteins and takes them to proteasomes, which break them down like a garbage disposal. If ubiquitin doesn't work or can't handle the waste clearance task, the damaged proteins clump together into protein aggregates. These clumps are found in the brain cells of people with Parkinson's, as well as those with Alzheimer's and Huntington's disease. Researchers suspect that protein clumping may contribute to cell death. Additional research is necessary to learn more about the relationship between the Lewy body, protein clumping, and Parkinson's disease.

While the precise cause of Parkinson's disease remains open to debate, researchers have learned a great deal about other factors that play a role in who tends to develop the disease. The following chapter looks at who is most vulnerable to Parkinson's disease, including the roles of genetics, gender, geography, and toxic and viral exposures.

2

Who Gets Parkinson's Disease?

Parkinson's disease has mystified medical experts for more than a century. Yes, doctors understand that the condition appears when the dopamine-producing cells of the substantia nigra die off, but they don't really understand why this happens or who is most vulnerable. Why would the disease affect one brother and not another? Why would one neighbor develop tremors and stiffness, leaving the others healthy and strong? It didn't make sense.

One hundred years ago, doctors assumed Parkinson's disease was an inherited disorder. While medical experts at the time didn't know anything about DNA and the genetic code, they didn't have a better explanation. If Parkinson's disease wasn't an inherited trait or an accident of birth, where did it come from?

The link between Parkinson's disease and environmental exposure took hold during World War I, when an outbreak of viral *encephalitis lethargica* (a form of sleeping sickness) caused a progressive illness very similar to Parkinson's disease. (The movie *Awakenings* depicts the experimental use of dopamine on these patients; the results were remarkable, albeit ultimately not permanent.) If a virus could cause this Parkinson's syndrome, could other environmental factors—such as viruses or chemical and heavy metal exposures—also cause the disease? Researchers found that Parkinson's disease was, in fact, more common among people who had experienced certain types of chemical exposures.

The importance of environmental exposures became glaringly apparent in the 1980s when a group of intravenous drug abusers in northern California developed symptoms of Parkinson's disease, including tremors, muscle rigidity, and bradykinesia. The autopsies of the victims who did not survive showed a complete loss of the dopamine-producing cells in the substantia nigra.

All of the affected people were using the street drug MPTP, a synthetic form of heroin. In the body, the drug MPTP is metabolized into MPP+, a toxin known to destroy dopamine-producing cells in the brain. This episode provided irrefutable evidence of a link between environmental exposure and the development of parkinsonian symptoms.

That was not, of course, the end of the story. At the same time, genetic researchers began to unlock the genetic code. Researchers identified several genes that increased the likelihood that a person would develop Parkinson's disease. In the early 1990s, Dr. Lawrence Golbe described a form of familial Parkinson's disease that affected a number of people in a family of Greek and Italian descent; by comparing the genes of various family members, researchers were able to identify genes that seemed linked to Parkinson's disease. Since then, several different genes have been identified indicating an increased risk of developing the disease.

So where are we now? Most researchers now believe that Parkinson's disease is caused by a complex relationship between a number of environmental and genetic factors. In other words, there does not appear to be any single agent that causes Parkinson's disease among all of those who are exposed, nor does there appear to be a purely genetic cause for Parkinson's disease that explains why some people develop the condition and others do not. Instead, we're left with a much more complicated picture that involves a combination of environmental or toxic exposures, nutritional deficiencies, immune system weaknesses, and genetic vulnerabilities that come together to trigger Parkinson's disease. Some combination of factors must be in place for a person to develop the disease.

▌ The Genetic Link

The genetic material that makes us who we are is stored in our chromosomes. Chromosomes consist of deoxyribonucleic acid (DNA), which in turn consists of genes, the blueprints for our inherited traits, such as eye color, height, and even our vulnerability to some illnesses, such as heart disease, some cancers, and type 2 diabetes, among others. In the fall of 2006, researchers at the National Institute of Aging and National Institute of Neurological Disorders and Stroke completed a study comparing blood samples of about 270 people with PD and the same number without PD. The results are inconclusive at this point, but the data should prove useful for future researchers.

When assessing whether a disease is inherited, researchers examine family medical history. (I was adopted at birth, but in adulthood I tracked down my birth mother, who did not have a family history of Parkinson's disease; the medical history of my birth father remains a mystery.) The genetic link is strongest with first-degree relatives: parents, siblings, and children. The larger the number of family members with the same medical condition, the greater the likelihood that a genetic factor is present.

The genetic influence among people with Parkinson's disease remains a topic of debate. Some experts estimate that only 10 to 15 percent of people with Parkinson's disease have a family member with the disease, indicating that the condition does not have a strong genetic influence. Other researchers, however, estimate that as many as 35 to 40 percent of people with Parkinson's disease have a first-degree relative who has the condition.

Determining which family members have the disease can be difficult because it can take many years for Parkinson's symptoms to be expressed and for the condition to be diagnosed. A majority of the dopamine-producing cells need to be destroyed before Parkinson's symptoms appear, so some researchers believe that many people have subclinical Parkinson's disease that is never diagnosed. If this is true, the importance of genetics may be underestimated because many more family members may have very mild forms of the disease that escape diagnosis.

Some families have an undeniable pattern of Parkinson's disease within the family tree. In these rare families, multiple family members across several generations have the disease. One of the most well known families with inherited Parkinson's disease is the Contursi family; 60 family members over five generations with the disease, according to research done by Dr. Golbe in 1990.

Autopsies of several family members showed the classic loss of dopamine cells and the presence of Lewy bodies. Later studies by Dr. Mihael Polymeropoulos in 1996 and 1997 identified a genetic mutation on a single chromosome that appeared to be the genetic cause of Parkinson's disease among these family members. At least five genes have been linked to Parkinson's disease, including alpha-synuclein, parkin, dardarin, ubiquitin carboxy-terminal hydrolase L1, and DJ–1. Researchers have found some of these genes to be dominant, and others recessive. (If a gene is dominant, a person needs to inherit only one gene from either parent to develop the disease; if a gene is recessive, a person needs to inherit the abnormal gene from both parents to develop the disease.) Other researchers have identified biomarkers that may be used in the future to help identify Parkinson's disease in its early stages based on a blood test.

Research on twins with Parkinson's disease has shown a difference between young-onset Parkinson's disease and the traditional form of the disease. The studies have shown little increased risk of one twin developing traditional Parkinson's disease, even when an identical twin has the disease, unless the illness occurred before age 50. The risk of one twin developing Parkinson's disease increased almost six times if the symptomatic twin showed signs of the disease before 50. This study suggests a greater genetic link in young-onset Parkinson's disease (discussed below), although additional research is necessary to learn more.

▮ Is Parkinson's Disease Inherited? ▮

The following chart, compiled by Dr. Jill Marjama-Lyons, is considered to be a good estimate of the risk of inheriting Parkinson's disease based on family history.

Person with Parkinson's Disease in Your Family	Chance of Getting Parkinson's Disease
None	1–2 percent, same as general population
Brother or sister	5–6 percent
One parent	10 percent
Parent and sibling	20–40 percent

As the table shows, even if some family members have Parkinson's disease, there is no reason to assume that other family members will develop it as well. The risk of developing Parkinson's disease increases with prevalence in a family, but most people will *not* develop the disease, even if other family members have it.

▎Beyond Genetics

In addition to the genetic vulnerabilities, other factors play an important role in who ultimately develops Parkinson's disease. Some of these factors include gender, age, geography, toxic exposures, viral exposures, estrogen deficiency, caffeine, nicotine, and nutrition.

Gender

Parkinson's disease is somewhat more common among men than women, a trend that holds true around the world. Researchers do not know whether this is due to some kind of protective effect of female hormones or men's greater exposure to environmental toxins through the work environment. Men tend to dominate the occupations that put them at risk for such exposure; on the other hand, teachers (a predominantly female occupation) have been placed on the list of occupations at higher risk of PD. As Michael and I have come in contact with thousands of people with Parkinson's worldwide, I have begun to question whether PD is in fact more prevalent in men; we see more and more women being stricken, especially with young-onset Parkinson's disease.

Age

The older you are, the greater your risk of developing Parkinson's disease, whether you are a man or woman. This is due to the natural degeneration of the dopamine-producing cells, as well as the fact that we are living longer. The incidence of Parkinson's disease is less than 10 per 100,000 per year for people under age 50, compared to more than 200 per 100,000 for people over age 80.

▌ Young-Onset Parkinson's Disease

Parkinson's disease is not, as I can testify, a disease of the elderly. While the majority of people with the disease are older, experts estimate that about 15 percent of the people with Parkinson's disease develop symptoms before age 50. However, the rate of young-onset Parkinson's disease is definitely on the rise. I believe this is due to a combination of better diagnosis and more exposure to toxins that have been found to contribute to PD. Those of us who develop the disease prior to age 55 are considered to have YOPD. Very rarely, people under age 21 develop the disease, which is then classified as juvenile-onset Parkinson's disease.

When actor Michael J. Fox announced that he had YOPD, the public—and many doctors—became aware for the first time that Parkinson's can strike people in their thirties and forties. There goes the stereotype of the gray-haired octogenarian stooped over, trembling, and shuffling across the room.

YOPD destroys the dopamine-producing cells in the brain, just as traditional Parkinson's disease does. There are, however, some important differences between the two.

▌ *Side effects from medication.* At first, younger people tend to respond better to dopamine-stimulating drugs than older people do. However, over time, people with young-onset Parkinson's tend to develop complications with the medicine, including wearing off (episodes when the medication suddenly stops working or wears off) and dyskinesia (unwelcome movements related to the drug). These problems with medication can appear within a month or a year of starting treatment. An estimated 55 percent of people with young-onset Parkinson's disease develop dyskinesia within one year of starting levodopa and 74 percent within three years, compared to 28 to 50 percent in three to five years among people with traditional Parkinson's disease.

▌ *Dystonia.* Limb dystonia is a cramping and "posturing" of muscles. This complication occurs in up to 43 percent of people with young-onset Parkinson's disease, compared to only 4 percent of people with traditional Parkinson's disease. Dystonia can become one of the more debilitating aspects of this disease, causing pain and the inability to function normally.

▌ *Mental changes.* It has been said that people with young-onset Parkinson's disease have less trouble with memory and cognitive problems than people with traditional Parkinson's disease. From our experience and contact with others with YOPD, this is not always the case. It is important to understand and begin to take steps to keep your mind sharp as early as possible. Almost every day I make an effort to work puzzles and math exercises; to be honest, I am deathly afraid of losing the ability to think for myself.

▌ *Slower progression.* Most experts agree that people with young-onset Parkinson's disease experience slower progression of the disease, compared to people with traditional Parkinson's disease. Many of us who suffer from the disease would dispute that. There are those of us, myself included, who have very rapid progression of their PD symptoms. Often, however, this progression will even out and slow down in later years.

Many people with YOPD have trouble getting an accurate diagnosis because their doctors don't consider the possibility that a young person can develop the disease. Doctors can have blinders on when it comes to Parkinson's disease, refusing to see what is in front of them because they cannot imagine an otherwise healthy person in their thirties coming down with this disease. Overcoming this prejudice is a matter of education.

This is one reason why the person with YOPD needs to become as knowledgeable as possible about the disease, including treatments and outreach. You must be your own team leader. You know what is going on inside your body. Ask questions and demand answers. Even after the diagnosis, most of us find that we have to find the right neurologist or movement-disorder specialist. Although the second neurologist I saw was outstanding, when I moved, it took me several tries to find the right doctor, one who had seen others with YOPD and understood my individual needs.

As discussed throughout the book, people with young-onset Parkinson's disease face some unique challenges. Many of us are diagnosed when we are just beginning to excel in our professions, raise our children, or take on mortgages and other long-term financial obligations. Sometimes we're still paying off our college loans at the same time we're learning that we have a lifelong chronic illness. The inherent unfairness of it all can feel overwhelming, and the thought of being sick for a lifetime can feel daunting. It is absolutely essential, in my opinion, that people with young-onset Parkinson's disease make an effort to develop a network of support so that they will not feel they are facing these challenges alone. The Parkinson's community is a diverse, supportive, empathetic group of people—young and old—who can walk with you on your journey of self-care and self-discovery.

Geography

Parkinson's disease is more prevalent in rural areas than urban areas, but the underlying reason for the difference is not clear. It could reflect differences in exposure to environmental toxins (such as pesticides) or access to health care, but researchers have not been able to firmly establish an explanation.

Environmental Exposures: Toxins

Parkinson's disease is more common among people in industrialized nations. Specific exposures that have been linked to Parkinson's disease include:

▎ *Pesticides.* Parkinson's disease is more prevalent among people who work in vegetable farming and drink well water. A laboratory study of rats exposed to rotenone, a chemical found in many pesticides, found that the animals developed rigidity and bradykinesia similar to that found in Parkinson's disease.

I grew up in California when the government sprayed for the Med fly. I can remember limiting outside activities on the spray days, and finding a film all over my car at the end of the day. A haze settled over the area. I knew we were being exposed to the pesticide, but I didn't imagine the potential harm.

When Michael was growing up, he and his friends used to ride their bikes behind the fogging trucks that released pesticides to kill the mosquitoes. Today, it's unimaginable that anyone would do this, but 30 years ago, most people assumed these pesticides were not harmful to humans. Studies have linked PD to exposure to the pesticides dieldrin and DDT, among others.

▌ *Paper mills and manufacturing plants.* People exposed to the chemicals used in paper production and manufacturing tend to have a higher than normal likelihood of developing Parkinson's disease. My ex-husband worked at a wood-processing plant in Tennessee, and he was exposed to myriad chemicals. He came home with formaldehyde, phenols, and other chemical residue on his clothes, which I then handled and washed. In addition, he worked at a textile mill, and the chemicals used there came home on his clothes and skin as well. Before that, I lived in West Virginia near a creosote plant. I can't prove any connection, but I suspect that my exposure to these chemicals may have contributed to my Parkinson's disease.

▌ *Heavy metals.* Occupational exposure to heavy metals—copper, lead, iron, manganese, and so forth—increases the risk of developing Parkinson's disease by up to 10 times compared to the normal population. In addition, the iron and aluminum content is much higher than normal in the brains of people with Parkinson's disease. It comes as no surprise that welders tend to have higher than average rates of PD. Other high-risk occupations include auto mechanics and those who serve in the military; Michael worked as a mechanic and he served in the Marines.

Gary, who was diagnosed at age 45, suspects that his Parkinson's disease could have been triggered by chemical and heavy-metal exposure as a child. "When I was growing up, I spent time with my grandfather, who did a lot of arc welding at his automotive repair shop," he said. "He also used chemical solvents to clean engine parts. To make matters worse, we lived in California near the orange groves, which were sprayed constantly. Who knows what was in the water table?"

Gary is the only person in his family who has developed PD, although he suspects his grandfather may have had symptoms that were never diagnosed. "My grandfather had a head bob," Gary said. "We don't know if it would have evolved into Parkinson's because he succumbed to cancer before we could find out."

▌ *Carbon monoxide.* People exposed to high levels of carbon monoxide, carbon disulfides, and other organic solvents have a greater incidence of Parkinson's disease. In one unusual case, a 13-year-old boy developed Parkinson's disease; he had experienced carbon monoxide poisoning when he was 8 years old.

It can be exquisitely difficult to prove a relationship between a toxic exposure and later development of Parkinson's disease, or any other health problem, for that matter. There is no test that can prove a causal link between an episode of chemical exposure and a disease that may not show up for years or decades later. The link between exposure and Parkinson's disease can be even more difficult to establish, since 60 to 70 percent of the dopamine-producing brain cells must be destroyed before symptoms appear.

Environmental Exposures: Viral Infections
As doctors learned during the outbreak of sleeping sickness during World War I, viral infections may also play a role in triggering

Parkinson's disease. At least 15 million people were infected with the virus, and of those about 6 million developed Parkinson's symptoms. (In fact, autopsies performed on some of the people with this disease found that they suffered from a viral brain infection that had similar symptoms but was not actually Parkinson's disease; the condition is technically referred to as post-encephalitic Parkinson's disease.)

Some researchers have considered an infectious link to Parkinson's disease, noting higher levels of certain antibodies in the cerebrospinal fluid of people with PD. They also suspect that the virus may cause inflammation in the brain, possibly damaging the dopamine-producing cells. On the other hand, Parkinson's disease doesn't follow the patterns of a spreading epidemic, so most researchers believe that other factors must also play an important role in determining who develops PD.

I had dengue fever when I was a teenager. It is contracted in the same way as malaria, through mosquito bites, and causes very high fever and delirium. It took more than a month for me to get back on my feet. Is there a connection to my PD? I don't know.

Low Levels of Estrogen

Some researchers believe that the female hormone estrogen may help protect against developing Parkinson's disease. The estrogen connection was supported by research published in the journal *Movement Disorders,* which compared the medical records of 72 women with Parkinson's disease and a group of women the same age who did not have the disease. The researchers found that the women who developed PD had three times the rate of hysterectomies, a higher rate of early menopause, and a lower rate of estrogen replacement therapy after menopause. This study suggests that estrogen may help to prevent or delay the onset of Parkinson's disease.

In my case, I suffered from polycystic ovary syndrome and endometriosis most of my adult life. I was unable to conceive children, and the condition went untreated for years. Once the condition was detected, I learned that my estrogen levels were lower than normal.

Caffeine

While caffeine is often blamed for negative health effects, it has been associated with a lower rate of Parkinson's disease. According to a study published in the *Journal of the American Medical Association*, the risk of developing Parkinson's disease is higher among people who did not drink coffee than it was among people who drank three cups (28 ounces) of caffeinated coffee daily. The findings were supported by other researchers who found that coffee drinkers developed Parkinson's disease eight years later than people who didn't drink coffee. This hasn't been true for Michael or me; we're both java hounds.

Now, these studies probably don't mean that caffeine—or some other ingredient in coffee—protects the brain from the ravages of Parkinson's disease. If you don't drink coffee, it probably doesn't make sense to brew a cup and try to pick up the habit. In addition, people who drink more than three or four cups daily often experience more severe tremor, nausea, and greater problems with insomnia. If you like to wake up to a morning cup of java, keep things in moderation, relax, and enjoy.

Nicotine

Cigarette smoking is harmful to your health. It contributes to heart disease, stroke, hypertension, lung cancer, and other cancers and health problems. Ironically, however, people who smoke cigarettes have lower rates of Parkinson's disease than those who don't smoke. For reasons that are not well understood, nicotine appears to protect the dopamine-producing cells in the brain. In laboratory research, nicotine has been shown to protect the brains of rats from cell death caused by exposure to the toxin MPTP. In human studies involving the nicotine patch, participants wearing the patch showed no improvement in motor symptoms compared to people with PD who did not wear the patch. The interaction between nicotine and Parkinson's disease remains under investigation.

I am a smoker—and I have been since before my PD was diagnosed—but I try to justify this vice by calling it a treatment for my PD. My doctor reminds me that this doesn't make sense; the health hazards far outweigh any possible benefits. Do as I say, not as I do: don't smoke.

"I am a smoker," said Marian, 60. "I could quit, but I find that my down time is more pronounced and my symptoms are more exaggerated when I don't smoke. Even my doctor jokes that I have the only disease that smoking is good for, but I know he's kidding. I don't want to live with Parkinson's only to die of lung cancer."

Diet and Nutrition

The relationship between diet and nutrition and Parkinson's disease remains controversial. Nothing you may eat—or fail to eat—has been definitively linked to PD, but some studies do suggest that diet may help to treat or prevent some cases of the disease. Specifically, diets rich in antioxidants—such as vitamin C, vitamin E, and beta-carotene—may help to reduce the levels of free radicals in the body, reducing the risk of developing Parkinson's disease. The importance of diet and nutritional supplements is discussed in detail in Chapter 8.

Clearly, Parkinson's disease is a multifaceted disease caused by a complex interaction of factors. For this reason, it is very difficult to identify who might be vulnerable to Parkinson's disease. It can also be very difficult to diagnose the disease, especially among people with young-onset Parkinson's disease. Chapter 3 describes some of the challenges doctors face when trying to diagnose the disease, and it outlines some of the steps your physician will have to take in order to accurately diagnose your condition.

3

Do You Have Parkinson's Disease?

For six years, Sarah, 59, suffered from various seemingly unrelated health concerns. Her handwriting became a "microscopic scribble" so small that no one in her office could read her written messages. Her right hand was bunched into a fist and she couldn't relax it. Her jaw locked and froze—a condition her doctor diagnosed as severe TMJ. Her boss told her she walked like an old lady. Her face became unexpressive. "My employees would say, 'You're staring at me like you're an owl,'" she said.

"When the tremors started and I had to have my friends write checks for me, I knew there was something terribly wrong," Sarah said. "Now I see that I had symptoms for six years, but the doctors tried to fix each symptom one at a time. All the pieces of the puzzle were there, but no one put it all together." After years of misdiagnosis, Sarah saw a movement-disorders specialist who recognized the classic symptoms of Parkinson's disease.

Parkinson's disease can be very difficult to diagnose. It involves a wide range of fickle symptoms that come and go without warning, and each person with the disease can show a somewhat different constellation of complaints. My diagnosis seemed obvious in hindsight; once I knew I had Parkinson's, all of those strange sensations I had been experiencing for years suddenly made sense.

I knew something was wrong before my tremor became evident and I developed my primary Parkinson's symptoms. I didn't know what was going on—and I never thought of Parkinson's disease—but for years before I was diagnosed I periodically felt a tickle in my fingers or a slight twitch in my right hand.

Like many other people with Parkinson's, I also experienced severe fatigue. At the time, I was attending weeklong horse shows with my daughter, and by the end of the week, I could barely stand. I felt shaky on the inside, my muscles ached, and sometimes my right arm would cramp up. I was also teaching, and almost every day I had to go to the school nurse and ask her to help me work out the cramp. My doctors tested for lupus and Lyme disease, but nothing explained what I was feeling.

In retrospect, it is clear that I was experiencing early symptoms of Parkinson's disease. Often months or years before the classic symptoms become obvious, someone with Parkinson's experiences some of the foreshadowing symptoms. These include:

- Fatigue
- Muscle aches
- Lack of coordination with motor tasks (such as buttoning, dressing, etc.)
- Poor balance
- Constipation
- Micrographia (small handwriting)
- Depression
- Decreased arm swing when walking
- Slow movement, almost as if you're moving under water
- A jackknife effect when you touch your forefinger and middle finger together

▌ Seborrheic dermatitis (red, scaly rash)
▌ Feeling something undefined is wrong with your health

I felt "off" for years before my final diagnosis, but my complaints were not severe enough to stop me from doing my daily activities. My symptoms continued to stump my rheumatologist, even though I kept feeling worse and worse. My doctor's assessment changed—and so did my own—when I developed my first classic Parkinson's symptom, a tremor in my right hand. At that point, my doctor began to consider that I could have Parkinson's disease.

Doctors—even excellent, well-intentioned, top-of-the-line neurologists—sometimes struggle with the diagnosis of Parkinson's disease because the symptoms can be intermittent and confused with symptoms of other diseases. As a rule, people with Parkinson's exhibit at least two of the classic motor symptoms of the disease—tremor, rigidity, and bradykinesia—but they often experience some of the other symptoms as well.

This chapter will describe the symptoms of Parkinson's disease—both the classic motor symptoms, as well as the other common signs—and it will discuss the process a physician goes through when making a clinical diagnosis. Keep in mind that not everyone with Parkinson's disease experiences every symptom—and not everyone with these symptoms has Parkinson's disease. You will need to be evaluated by a neurologist or Parkinson's disease specialist to confirm any diagnosis.

James, 51, had some muscle weakness and found it difficult to walk up stairs, but he attributed his fatigue to growing older and not exercising enough. When he developed pain in his chest, he sought medical care. "It took seven doctors fourteen months to figure out what was going on," he said. "Three out of four doctors told me it was anxiety and gave me drugs for that. Finally, by the end of the fourteen months, I developed a tremor and had such weakness that I had real trouble walking. I went to the library and checked the *Physicians' Desk Reference*. I determined I had either multiple sclerosis or Parkinson's. Turns out the ongoing pain in my chest was my diaphragm spasming."

While some of the behaviors can seem strange or frightening, don't worry: they can be controlled with medication. Over the years, I have had firsthand experience with just about every Parkinson's side effect, but they do not dominate my daily life, and they do not define who I am.

▮ The Three Classic Parkinson's Symptoms

As we've said, at the most basic level, Parkinson's disease affects the dopamine levels in the brain, causing problems with motor function or movement of the body. While movement can include everything from walking to the mailbox to swallowing your morning coffee, the three classic movement problems that define Parkinson's disease are tremor, rigidity, and bradykinesia (slowness of movement). Different people exhibit different symptoms: some people have tremors and problems with rigidity, while others might have bradykinesia and rigidity but no tremor at all.

Symptoms of Parkinson's disease usually show up on one side of the body. Over time, most people develop symptoms on both sides, but for most of us one side remains more symptomatic than the other.

The symptoms of Parkinson's disease can be quite unpredictable. They vary from hour to hour and day to day. Many people with Parkinson's have good days, when they have very few active symptoms, but inevitably they also experience bad days when they tremble and freeze throughout the day. Most people with Parkinson's find that when their medication is in balance, their movements are basically normal—and, conversely, when their medication wears off or when they are tired or stressed, the Parkinson's symptoms become more active. When I'm exhausted or unhappy, my body lets me know by making my Parkinson's worse; this is a way of reminding me that I need to slow down and take care of myself.

Gary, 50, experienced many minor symptoms that went unnoticed by most people, although his wife noticed that something was wrong. "I had problems with my gait; I took short steps and my arms didn't swing much when I walked. I lacked expression in my face, and I had lots of mood swings. My wife noticed the symptoms before anyone else did, and she noticed that they seemed to come and go."

Tremor

Tremor—the most obvious and well known of the Parkinson's disease symptoms—is another word for a trembling or shaking of the body. Mine started in my right arm, but it can also show up in the leg or jaw. Many people think of tremor as a classic symptom of Parkinson's disease, but as many as one out of three people with Parkinson's do not have tremor. To make things even more complicated, in a rare variation of PD called *tremor-predominant Parkinson's,* a person has tremors but no other symptoms.

There are several types of tremor:

- *Rest tremor.* This tremor occurs when the limb—usually the fingers, wrist, or arm—is relaxed and not in use. It stops when the limb is moved.
- *Postural tremor.* This tremor occurs when an arm or leg is held out against gravity, such as when holding a newspaper or book while reading.
- *Action tremor.* This tremor occurs when the limb is in use, such as when putting on makeup or eating with a knife and fork.
- *Pill-rolling tremor.* This tremor involves rolling the thumb against the index finger, as if rolling a pill. (This was one of the first symptoms I showed when my Parkinson's moved to my left side.)

Your doctor should always evaluate possible tremor in three ways—at rest, with arms and legs extended, and when the limbs are in use.

Rigidity

Rigidity is a tightening or stiffening of the muscles. Typically, our muscles work in opposing pairs—the bicep paired with the tricep, for example—and one muscle contracts as the other relaxes. When someone has Parkinson's disease, the communication between the opposing muscles can be disturbed, and one set of muscles tenses, causing stiffness.

There are two basic types of rigidity: lead-pipe rigidity (the body won't move; it's stiff, like a lead pipe) and cogwheel rigidity (the body moves in a jerky motion, similar to the cogs in a wheel). In both types of rigidity, the body does not move smoothly, and there can be a great deal of pain.

Some people with Parkinson's have severe rigidity, while others don't experience it at all. My rigidity started early, but I didn't recognize what it was. My legs felt very stiff, they hurt, and they didn't operate right. Was I overusing them—or was I out of shape? Did I need to rest, or did I need to get more exercise?

Typically, rigidity occurs more on one side than on the other and involves the arms, legs, neck, and back. Once I experienced a bout of full-body rigidity: I couldn't move for 45 minutes. It was as if my entire body was tied up in a knot. I sat until the episode passed, and then I was gradually able to move again.

Bradykinesia

Bradykinesia is a general term referring to slowness of movement or speech. The term *akinesia* refers to absence of movement, which can also be a sign of Parkinson's disease; in most cases, akinesia shows up as an arm that does not swing when you walk or a similar inability to move voluntarily.

Most people with Parkinson's disease experience some type of bradykinesia, which can be expressed in a number of ways—from freeze attacks to difficulty dressing, from difficulty walking to difficulty swallowing. These symptoms will be discussed in greater detail in the "Common Symptoms" section on page 37, but they can be considered expressions of bradykinesia.

The symptoms of bradykinesia come and go, but when they are active, the person may feel weakness, although the muscles are completely normal. Parkinson's disease affects the communication between the brain and the muscles, creating slowness and stiffness, but the muscles themselves are healthy and strong (see Chapter 7).

Balance: A Fourth Symptom

Another very common symptom of Parkinson's disease is postural instability or problems with balance. While this is not considered one of the major motor symptoms (in part because so many other conditions can cause balance problems, including aging), many people with Parkinson's have trouble with their balance. I have been known to fall out of chairs or stumble when standing. Often it feels like it's happening in slow motion; I can feel myself falling, so I have time to catch myself or ease myself down without injury. About two years into my Parkinson's symptoms, however, I did fall and break my arm.

I couldn't pass a roadside sobriety test: I can't walk a straight line. In technical terms, people with Parkinson's sometimes propulse, meaning we lean too far forward, increasing the risk of falling. (We also tend to retropulse, or move backward, when standing up from sitting in a chair.) Sometimes we hunch forward, also contributing to our balance problems.

James, 51, has actually been pulled over by the police, under suspicion of driving under the influence.

One night I was dyskinetic while I was driving. I was hugging the line, weaving a bit. It was closing time at the bars, and I was pulled over. I hadn't been drinking—I almost never drink at all anymore—but my speech was slurred and I was shaking and looking nervous.

I was stopped by the police, and I showed my medic alert card, which declares, "I'm not intoxicated; I have Parkinson's disease. Please call my family or physician for help." I call it my Get Out of Jail Free card. The officer read it and said, "Okay, I understand. My grandfather has Parkinson's disease."

He didn't smell any alcohol on my breath, and I passed the breathalyzer test, of course. I turned the episode into an educational opportunity. I knew what the officer was seeing, and frankly, I would have done the same thing.

Common Symptoms

Parkinson's disease can express itself in a number of ways. The following is an A-to-Z list of common symptoms:

▌ *Autonomic nervous system changes.* The autonomic nervous system controls your heart rate, blood pressure, body temperature, digestive tract, and other involuntary nervous systems response. Some people with Parkinson's disease have trouble with their autonomic responses, contributing to a range of secondary complications. For example, my body isn't very good at regulating heat: I'm always hot, even when everyone else in the room is chilled. Michael, on the other hand, is often cold—but, fortunately for us, opposites attract.

▌ *Breathing difficulty.* Fortunately, it doesn't happen too often, but sometimes people with Parkinson's disease develop shortness of breath. They can breathe 20 to 24 times a minute, twice as fast as a normal, relaxed person. This can be a frightening symptom, and a person with breathing problems should always see a specialist to make sure there are no heart or lung problems.

▌ *Constipation.* Slow bowel movements are common in people with Parkinson's disease. If a high-fiber diet and regular exercise don't help, talk to your doctor.

▌ *Depression.* Depression occurs in about half of all people with Parkinson's disease. Depression is discussed in greater detail in Chapter 11.

▌ *Difficulty with fine-motor activities.* Tasks that require fine-motor coordination—such as buttoning, shaving, putting on makeup, tying shoes, picking up small objects—can be difficult or impossible for people with Parkinson's. Velcro will become your new best friend.

▌ *Difficulty initiating movement.* Many people with PD have trouble starting a movement, such as rolling over in bed, climbing out of a car, rising from a chair, or walking. It can feel as if you're stuck: your brain says go, but your feet say stop. This is called *start hesitancy,* and it usually lasts just a few minutes. (Tips on overcoming start hesitancy are discussed in Chapter 13.)

▌ *Dyskinesia.* This term describes a type of irregular, writhing movements; it is not a symptom of Parkinson's disease, but rather a side effect of the long-term use of carbidopa-levodopa. If the movements are fast, they are called *chorea;* if the movements are somewhat slow, they are called *athetosis;* if they are very slow—almost a posturing of the limb or body—they are called *dystonia.* I've had dystonias that felt like full-body cramps, and one that required medication so that I could release myself from the fetal position. Some people develop dyskinesia when they have too much dopamine; others when they have too little.

▌ *Dysphagia or difficulty swallowing.* For some people, the problem may be mild: difficulty swallowing large bites or sticky foods like caramel or peanut butter. For others, like me, it can involve swallowing almost anything, including water. I've had situations when my throat muscles have closed up on nothing, and I begin to choke. My lips turn blue, and all I can do is try to calm myself and relax. This is one of the most difficult symptoms for me.

▮ *Fainting and light-headedness.* Many people with PD feel light-headed or faint when they stand up. This can be a side effect caused by Parkinson's medications, or it can be caused by changes in the involuntary nervous system.

▮ *Freezing.* As the name implies, freezing occurs when someone with Parkinson's abruptly stops walking without warning. It often happens when trying to pass through doorways or when making a turn while walking. Freeze attacks typically last a few seconds or several minutes, although they can go on much longer. Sometimes people need to take several extra steps, as if turning on a square, rather than simply turning in one smooth movement; this is called *turning en bloc.* Sometimes I take a step or two, and then it feels like my foot is glued to the floor. (Tips on overcoming this symptom are described in Chapter 13.)

James has had difficulty freezing in public places. "About a half dozen times, I've frozen in public places like the local convenience store," he said. "I can't leave the counter. I turn to go and I can't move. Sometimes I can't talk, all I can do is bat my eyes.

"The longest I have frozen is four hours. That was frightening. I sense everything that's going on, but I can't move," James said. "It hurts. One time I was fishing on the bank of a pond. I was getting up to leave and I froze. It was dusk when I froze, and I couldn't leave until eleven P.M."

▮ *Hallucinations and delusions.* Visual hallucinations (seeing things that aren't there) and delusions (believing things that aren't true) can present themselves as Parkinson's symptoms. This type of cognitive problem usually does not occur until the disease is quite advanced. In some cases, these problems are related to side effects from various medications.

▌*Hypophonia.* Sometimes people with Parkinson's disease lose the volume and clarity of their voice. Some people find that their voice becomes soft and raspy. I tend to overcompensate to the point of almost yelling, although other times I mumble or can't get enough air out to make my voice heard.

▌*Masked face.* This refers to a lack of facial expression in some people with Parkinson's disease. It can be severe—like a blank stare—or just a joyless expression. I can laugh and smile, but sometimes I forget that my emotions aren't evident. My daughter once asked me, "Why aren't you ever happy?" I told her, "I may not be smiling on the outside, but I'm smiling on the inside."

▌*Micrographia.* This symptom is characterized by small handwriting; it can be mild or so severe that the writing becomes illegible. I tend to write like I'm in kindergarten, especially if I have to write a lot, so this is not my most debilitating symptom. Other people with Parkinson's have a lot of trouble with handwriting. "My handwriting is often illegible," said Lila, 49, "and it is hard for me to fill out forms. It irritates me."

▌*Numbness.* Sometimes people with Parkinson's disease experience numbness, tingling, and pain in their feet and hands. This condition, called *paresthesia,* may be linked to rigidity. It can be confused with other medical problems, such as peripheral neuropathy and arthritis.

▌*Olfactory changes.* Sometimes people with PD develop a decline in their sense of smell. Often I say to Michael, "Do you smell that? What is it?" He can rarely recognize what I'm talking about.

▌*Sexual difficulty and impotence.* Both men and women with Parkinson's disease can develop decreased libido—perhaps due to low dopamine levels—as well as difficulty achieving orgasm.

▌*Short-term memory problems.* Memory problems don't occur in early Parkinson's disease, but some cognitive problems often appear as the disease progresses. I used to teach higher math, and yet I remember sitting down to balance my checkbook and forgetting how to add and subtract. I looked at the numbers, but I had no idea what to do. I sometimes forget words in the middle of a sentence. If the problem becomes severe enough, it is classified as dementia. The condition is actually bradyphrenia, or slowed thinking; in other words, the person comes up with the correct response, but it takes a while. Unfortunately, it affects about one out of three people with Parkinson's disease.

▌*Siallorhea or excessive salivation.* When the swallowing reflex slows due to Parkinson's disease, a person can develop siallorhea, or excessive salivation. The saliva pools in the mouth and occasionally spills out in a puddle of drool. No, it's not pretty; sometimes I feel like I should carry around a bucket. I drool at night, so I wake up with a soaking wet face and pillow. While the problem is embarrassing, it can be dangerous if you aspirate saliva (breathe saliva into the lungs); this can cause pneumonia.

▌*Skin problems.* People with Parkinson's disease sometimes have seborrhea (a red rash), or scaling, flaking, or oily skin, especially on the face and forehead.

▌*Sleep problems.* I often feel that I haven't had a good night's sleep in 15 years. Many people with Parkinson's disease have trouble falling asleep, staying asleep, waking early, or waking in the night to use the bathroom. These problems are exacerbated by side effects from medications, depression, and a tendency to have little time in the deepest stages of sleep. Often people wake up with a restless feeling known as *akathisia;* relief only comes when you surrender to the sensation and walk or march around. Sometimes people develop restless-leg syndrome, a creeping sensation in the legs at night. I sometimes pace at night to wear myself out, only to find that the sensation returns as soon as my head hits the pillow. (Rest is discussed in greater detail in Chapter 10.)

▌*Urinary problems.* Difficulty urinating, frequent urination, urgent urination, nighttime urination, and incontinence can occur in people with Parkinson's disease. The problem can have its origins in the communication of the signals within the body; sometimes the Parkinson's symptoms—such as slow walking—can make it difficult to get to the bathroom in time.

▌ *Vision problems.* Blurry vision and jerky eye movements can occur with Parkinson's disease. I have trouble seeing at night, but my vision is usually clear during the day. People with Parkinson's should have annual eye exams.

▌ *Walking or gait problems.* Most people with Parkinson's disease have some trouble with walking, including walking slowly, dragging one leg, shuffling, or taking tiny steps. Sometimes there's a decrease in how much they can swing their arms on one side, contributing to balance problems. Another gait problem is *festation*, the tendency to take fast, small forward steps. It can also look like the person is running, taking small steps without lifting his legs. The person isn't trying to take baby steps, but when he starts to take a full step, somewhere between raising his foot and lowering it, his brain short-circuits and shortens the stride to only a few inches. If this happens to you, try not to worry about it: you'll get where you're going, it just may take a little longer.

▌ *Weight loss.* Unexplained weight loss occurs in a small percentage of people with PD. If you lose weight, work with your doctor to determine whether the change is due to depression or another medical problem; you don't want to allow your Parkinson's symptoms to blind you to other possible health problems.

Don't feel intimidated by the possible symptoms of Parkinson's disease. Symptoms vary from person to person, and day to day. A bothersome symptom may appear one day and then disappear forever. You should, however, keep track of the symptoms you experience, so that you can report them to your doctor, who may be able to recommend treatment. If you have not yet been definitively diagnosed with Parkinson's disease, careful reporting of your symptoms can help your doctor reach a diagnosis.

▮ Can Parkinson's Alter Vision and Touch? ▮

Although Parkinson's disease is considered a movement disorder, recent research indicates that it may also cause abnormalities in touch and vision. Researchers at Emory University Health Sciences Center used functional magnetic resonance imaging (MRI) technology to observe brain activity in people with Parkinson's during tactile-ability tests. They found that the study participants with PD had much less activity in the sensory areas of the brain than people without PD.

The study indicates that the boundaries between touch and vision and sensation and movement may be linked in a way the scientists did not appreciate previously. What does this mean for the day-to-day experience of someone living with PD? It may be important as physical therapists and Parkinson's researchers work to design new strategies for treatment and rehabilitation. It may also help you forgive yourself if you've been known to drop things or fling them when you have tremors. You're not clumsy; it's the Parkinson's.

▮ How Do You Know If You Have Parkinson's Disease?

Parkinson's disease is notoriously difficult to diagnose. In fact, most people with PD have symptoms for about five years before they are correctly diagnosed. Most of us end up consulting a number of doctors and specialists before we find someone able to offer an accurate diagnosis, not because we haven't been seeing good doctors, but because diagnosing Parkinson's disease involves a process of elimination. Your doctor can't accurately diagnose your condition until he or she rules out a number of other possible causes of your symptoms, and that typically involves lots of tests and physical exams with lots of neurologists and rheumatologists and other specialists.

This one-more-test, one-more-referral process can make you weary, I know. My hope is that by understanding what your doctor is doing and why, you may be able to feel less frustrated by the process. This section will describe the steps your doctor is likely to take in order to arrive at a final diagnosis.

▌The Process of Elimination

Diagnosing Parkinson's is so tricky because there are no definitive diagnostic tests for the disease. Your doctor can't order a blood test or a brain scan or an X-ray that will come back with a firm diagnosis because the region of the brain that produces dopamine is so small that most scanning equipment can't detect the microscopic changes that take place in the early stages of Parkinson's disease. (In fact, the only confirmation of diagnosis can be performed after death, when doctors can examine the substantia nigra for signs of decay.)

That's not to say that doctors don't use lots of high-tech testing while diagnosing Parkinson's disease. Most doctors prescribe CAT scans and MRIs, but these tests are typically used to rule out other disorders that could be causing similar symptoms. PET (positron emission tomography) scans and SPECT (single photon emission computed tomography) scans use radioactive compounds to measure blood flow and dopamine activity in the brain, but the equipment is not widely available, and it is very expensive. PET scans and SPECT scans are not currently used as diagnostic tools, but rather as screening tests for people who may have Parkinson's-plus syndromes.

Instead, your doctor has to do detective work. This is basically a three-step process.

Step 1: Assess the Symptoms

To diagnose Parkinson's disease, a doctor—preferably a neurologist or Parkinson's disease specialist—must review the patient's detailed medical history and perform a complete physical exam. The doctor should consider all the possible Parkinson's symptoms, including those described earlier in this chapter. Too often, some doctors dismiss PD as a diagnosis if a patient does not have a tremor. However, as mentioned earlier, about one out of three people with Parkinson's do not experience tremors.

Step 2: Consider All Possible Diagnoses

After collecting your report of symptoms, your doctor needs to consider whether or not you could have another disease or condition. In the early stages of the disease, it can be difficult to distinguish between Parkinson's and other conditions. Are you moving slowly because you have rigidity due to Parkinson's disease or arthritis due to old age? Is your hand trembling due to a benign tremor, or do you have Parkinson's disease?

To make this determination, your doctor should consider the possibility that you have another condition with symptoms similar to those of Parkinson's disease, such as the following:

▌ *Aging.* Most people slow down as they grow older. They often walk more slowly and deliberately, become forgetful, or experience difficulty with balance. Some older people develop an essential tremor (discussed below), which can easily be confused with a tremor of Parkinson's disease.

▌ *Arthritis.* Arthritis involves bone and joint pain; it can cause some people to walk slowly, lose motor coordination, or stoop over. It differs from Parkinson's disease in these ways:

- Arthritis can be confirmed with X-rays and blood tests.
- Arthritis causes joint pain, not muscle pain.
- The pains of Parkinson's disease don't respond to the medications used to treat arthritis.
- Arthritis does not cause a tremor, and muscle tone remains normal.

▌ *Depression.* Depression can cause slow movement, stooped posture, weight loss, and other common symptoms of Parkinson's disease. In addition, depression often coexists with Parkinson's disease, making diagnosis more difficult. Your doctor needs to perform a physical evaluation to determine if you show other signs of Parkinson's disease. (Depression is discussed in greater detail in Chapter 11.)

▌ *Essential tremor.* Many people—including doctors—confuse essential tremor with parkinsonian tremor. Essential tremor is about 10 times more common than Parkinson's disease. People with essential tremor do not exhibit any other symptoms of Parkinson's disease, such as rigidity, bradykinesia, or problems with balance. Essential tremor is usually an action tremor that occurs on both the left and right sides (it is bilateral), while Parkinsonian tremor usually appears at rest and only on one side. A correct diagnosis is important because essential tremor and Parkinson's disease do not respond to the same treatments.

▌ *Stroke.* In some cases, people with Parkinson's disease are misdiagnosed as having suffered a stroke because they present symptoms on one side of the body. (This is most common when the person does not experience tremor.) In stroke, symptoms typically appear quickly—within hours—while PD symptoms develop gradually, over many years. The brain scans of people with PD are normal, whereas evidence of stroke shows up in both CAT scans and MRIs. People who have suffered a stroke also fail to respond to treatment with the medications used to treat Parkinson's disease.

Step 3: Try a Trial Dose of Medication

If the symptoms tend to indicate Parkinson's disease, a doctor typically prescribes a trial dose of dopamine-stimulating medication. If the patient's condition improves, he or she is considered to have Parkinson's disease; if the patient does not improve, the doctor must consider another diagnosis.

I distinctly remember when I began taking medication to find out if I had Parkinson's disease. On the one hand, I felt relieved to be free of my symptoms and to finally have a diagnosis—a disease with a name—after so many years of searching. On the other hand, I was devastated to have been diagnosed with Parkinson's disease, a chronic, lifelong disease that promised to progress over the years. That said, I believe it's easier to fight the enemy you know than the enemy you don't.

Lila, who was diagnosed with Parkinson's at age 42, remembers the moment she learned she had PD.

I had no energy and I walked in a slump. I didn't swing my arms. Before long, I walked on tiptoes, taking tiny baby steps. I took muscle relaxants for the cramps and to loosen my muscles, but nothing helped.

I went to a psychiatrist, and he put me on an antidepressant. Then I got another drug to help me sleep, but I knew something else was wrong. He gave me another drug. In the morning, instead of being unable to walk, I got up and danced around the room. I felt like a new person. I called the doctor and said, "I'm a poster child for this medicine."

It was Sinemet.

When I went to see him, he told me I have Parkinson's disease. I was overwhelmed. It was the beginning of my life with Parkinson's, but I felt like it was the end of my life as me.

Part 2 of this book will describe the drug therapy and surgical options considered part of conventional treatment for Parkinson's disease. In addition, it will outline factors you should consider when finding a physician to work with you as you take the steps necessary to live well with Parkinson's disease.

▌ Secondary Parkinson's Disease ▌

In some situations, a person exhibits all the symptoms of Parkinson's disease, but the condition is a secondary response to another problem. Most secondary Parkinson's disease is caused by side effects of medications that block the dopamine activity of the brain, including some antipsychotic and antinausea drugs. Secondary Parkinson's disease caused by medication typically clears up within six months of discontinuing the drug.

Secondary Parkinson's disease can also be caused by head trauma, stroke, or brain tumors located near the dopamine-producing region of the brain. The boxer Muhammad Ali suffers from secondary Parkinson's disease. In these cases, the Parkinson's symptoms tend to be irreversible.

PART TWO

Traditional Medical Care

4

Drugs for Parkinson's Disease

When Marian was 52, she thought she had multiple sclerosis. She was so weak she couldn't push herself up to get out of bed in the morning. Her body trembled; she couldn't raise her arms or stand erect. "I felt my whole body was lead," she said. "I couldn't move."

Marian was referred to a neurologist who wasn't sure if she had MS or Parkinson's disease. "My doctor gave me the miracle drug—Sinemet—and within two days I felt a change," Marian said. "I felt like I was nineteen again. I was cured."

Marian enjoyed a couple of weeks of strength, and then returned to her doctor. "Two weeks later when I went back, the doctor said, 'This proves one hundred percent that you have Parkinson's.' Then he said I couldn't have any more of the drug. He said it wouldn't last but a few years, so I should save it for later, when my symptoms would be worse.

"I begged for the drug. What good would it be years from now if I lost all desire to do a lot of the things I want to do now? I pleaded, but he wouldn't give it to me."

Instead, Marian began the classic drug regimen for Parkinson's: drugs known as dopamine agonists, which directly stimulate the receptors in the nerves in the brain that normally would be stimulated by dopamine. Unlike levodopa, dopamine agonists are not converted into dopamine when they enter the body, but they behave like dopamine. When dopamine agonists lose their power to control the symptoms of Parkinson's disease, doctors prescribe Sinemet—a combination of the drugs levodopa and carbidopa. Levodopa is in a class of medications called central nervous system agents; it is converted into dopamine in the brain. Carbidopa is in a class of medications called decarboxylase inhibitors; it prevents levodopa from being broken down before it reaches the brain.

Over time—typically a period of several years—this medication also loses its ability to tame the tremors and other symptoms of Parkinson's; or a person develops unpleasant side effects, including dyskinesia (uncontrolled movements). At this point, people with Parkinson's must either experiment with changing their doses or they may consider surgery (see Chapter 5).

Since the medications tend to provide relief for a period of years, the problems with "medication fatigue" tend to be greater in people who are diagnosed at younger ages. Older people often find that medications can control their symptoms without problems or complications throughout their lives.

This chapter will examine the major classes of Parkinson's drugs. It's important for you to understand all of the different medications so you can know how to use them effectively. Many of them can have unpleasant side effects. I find that if a medication tends to make me ill, I take the first dose at 5 A.M. with a sip of cola to coat my stomach. Then I go back to sleep. That way, I have some medication working in my system when I wake up in the morning.

I really hate being dependent on drugs. I hate feeling tied to my medicine bottle, but I panic when I look into the bottle and see that I'm down to just two or three pills. There are times I want to take my entire bag of meds and throw it in the Gulf of Mexico, but I know that without my drugs I would be a nonfunctioning human being. In those moments I try to remind myself to be grateful that I have so many medications available to me, and that with drugs I can outsmart my Parkinson's, at least for a little while.

Lila, who was diagnosed with PD at age 42, understands. "I fake it to make it," she said. "Everywhere I go, I take my bag of meds. Sometimes I don't want to think about it, but when I'm out and my symptoms come on, I need to have what I need to handle things."

▋ Understanding Parkinson's Medications

Most Parkinson's medications either replace missing dopamine or allow the body to use whatever dopamine it has more effectively. For any of the medications to work, they must be absorbed from the gastrointestinal tract and move into the blood, which takes them to the brain. Blood can't flow freely into the brain; substances must cross the blood-brain barrier, a filter designed to protect the delicate brain from any potential contaminants. In addition, pure dopamine can't cross into the brain; instead, it must be delivered as levodopa. For years, levodopa was the drug of choice for Parkinson's disease, but researchers improved on it further by combining it with carbidopa, another drug that helps prevent the breakdown of levodopa in the body. Sinemet—the gold standard for Parkinson's treatment—is a combination of levodopa and carbidopa.

With any medication for Parkinson's, talk to your doctor about how to dose the medication. I know some people who wake up in the middle of the night to take a dose of their medications; others go from night until morning with no additional medication.

Pay attention to what you're feeling. Doctors only know what they read; you live with Parkinson's every day and you know what the medication is doing to your body. You'll probably need to try different medications at different doses before you find the right "cocktail" to control your symptoms—and then, just when you think you've got it worked out, things will change. Some days your medication just won't work right. Be prepared for these inevitable ups and downs and try not to let them frustrate you. Parkinson's disease can be temperamental, and you're going to have to adjust to the constant changes in your body.

▌ Dopamine Agonists

Dopamine agonists include apomorphine (Apokyn), bromocriptine (Parlodel), pergolide (Permax), pramipexole (Mirapex), and ropinirole (Requip).

Many neurologists first prescribe a dopamine agonist for the treatment of Parkinson's, especially in patients under age 70. These medications stimulate the dopamine receptors in the brain; they are structurally similar to dopamine, so they can bind with the dopamine receptors. They don't work quite as well as levodopa itself, but they do help ease Parkinson's symptoms. In addition, by starting with dopamine agonists, the person with Parkinson's can delay the use of levodopa, in essence saving this drug for later use, if needed.

Studies have shown that dopamine agonists can be as effective as levodopa in controlling PD symptoms, with fewer motor side effects. Most studies have found that dopamine agonists produce about half the rate of motor side effects as levodopa.

Unlike the other agonists, which are taken orally, apomorphine must be injected. This drug is often used for sudden relief when other medications don't work or when they wear off too soon.

Dopamine agonists can cause edema (swelling), psychosis, drowsiness or sudden sleep, as well as nausea and vomiting. I had terrible trouble with nausea and vomiting when I first went on Requip; I also couldn't think straight. The side effects went away as I adjusted to the drug, but it was quite unpleasant at first.

Gary, a 50-year-old man from Houston, experiences problems with sudden sleep when taking dopamine agonists. "When the medication starts to work, it makes you extremely drowsy," he said. "I can usually fight it. If I'm moving, I can work through it, but if I'm sitting down, sleep can sneak up on me.

"I have to be careful driving or I'll have a narcoleptic attack," Gary said. "When I take long trips, I cut back on the dose for a day or two. I once swerved off the highway when driving. I'm lucky; I came out unscathed."

Some people also report trouble with compulsions or impulse control when on these medications, especially Mirapex (see box). Lila, 49, has experienced some minor compulsions. "I brush my teeth five times a day, and I wash my hands ten or fifteen times," she said. "I'm real particular about my laundry, and, to be honest, I want to buy a new pair of shoes every time I go to the store."

"I Just Couldn't Stop"

Gary was 45 when he was diagnosed with Parkinson's disease. While taking the dopamine agonist Mirapex, he experienced shopping, gambling, and sexual compulsions, all well-known side effects of the medication. This is his story:

I'm not an addictive personality, but I've had my share of trouble with Mirapex. I had been collecting die-cast toy cars with my sons. We were very selective and knowledgeable about collecting them, choosing only cars of good quality and value.

When I was diagnosed with Parkinson's disease, I became obsessed with these toy cars. I bought anything; they didn't have to be collectible or hard to find. I couldn't drive by a toy store or Wal-Mart without stopping. I couldn't leave the store without buying at least one, even if I already had the same one at home. I went to twenty-four-hour stores that would get their shipments in overnight. My wife—my ex-wife—would come home every day and find a bag of toys on the kitchen counter.

I have ten thousand of these cars.

It all seemed perfectly reasonable at the time. Part of me knew they weren't valuable, but I couldn't stop myself. It's like I knew and I didn't know what I was doing at the same time.

I was eventually able to figure out the compulsion. I saw that what I was doing was lunacy. I am still a member of a car-collector club, but I don't go into stores. Sometimes I go over and take a look, but it's no longer a compulsive disorder.

I also came close to having a gambling disorder. I am familiar with gaming and I really like to throw the dice. That was my game of choice. I got a little out of control. I was gambling money that was earmarked to pay bills. I had to get into my credit.

That time, I was aware of the compulsion. It was like getting drunk—I lost my mind, but the next day I felt like I had a hangover, and I'd say to my wife, "Why did I do that?"

Now, I stay away from casinos.

With each of the compulsions, I feel like I have an angel on one shoulder and the devil on the other.

> *I've also struggled with a compulsion for hypersexuality. I've found myself in situations after my divorce when I've wondered, "What am I doing? This isn't me." I try not to be a player anymore, but I'm still a young man.*
>
> *The Mirapex is a boon and a bane. I need the drug to function physically, but it also makes the pleasure center in my brain say, "It's time to have fun." This has been a huge struggle. It's a pain in the butt to deal with all of these side effects, but I have to do it.*

▌ Levodopa-Carbidopa

Levodopa-carbidopa drugs include Sinemet, Atamet, and Parcopa.

Levodopa can pass from the bloodstream into the brain, where it is converted into dopamine. It is the gold standard for the treatment of Parkinson's disease, and has been for nearly 50 years. Carbidopa helps to keep the levodopa from breaking down before it reaches the brain, and it minimizes nausea and vomiting associated with the medication.

The drug usually kicks in about 20 to 40 minutes after taking it, and the benefit lasts two to four hours. That said, after a few years, some people experience "wearing off," in which the medicine doesn't seem to do much or stops working entirely. Some people also have on-off experiences with the drug: the medicine works one minute but not the next. In those cases, there's little to do but wait until it's time for another dose, although that's not always easy.

Levodopa-carbidopa is available in immediate-release, controlled-release, and extended-release formulas to minimize off time. Some people swear by the immediate-release Sinemet, claiming it is the only way they can get moving in the mornings; others rely on the extended-release pills, noting that the more gradual release of the medicine helps their mobility if they have to get up in the middle of the night to go to the bathroom. There is no formula that works best for everyone; trial and error is the best way to find the medicine or combination of medicines that works best for you.

Levodopa is an amino acid that must be absorbed through the wall of the intestines. Eating protein at the same time as taking levodopa will interfere with the absorption of the drug because the protein and the levodopa depend on the same transport system in the intestine. Bottom line: wait at least one-half hour after taking the pill before eating—or wait one hour after eating before taking the pill—to maximize the effectiveness of the drug.

Levodopa-carbidopa can cause nausea and vomiting, as well as low blood pressure (especially when standing), hallucinations, paranoia, sleepiness, and compulsive behavior. Long-term use of levodopa can cause dyskinesia—uncontrolled writhing and twitching—in 50 to 80 percent of people with PD. (Dyskinesia comes from the Latin root *dys,* meaning "not correct," and *kinesia,* meaning "movement.") In most people, dyskinesia does not appear until after three to five years of treatment, and can often take several years to become disabling.

Most people who develop dyskinesia have problems when they have too much levodopa (known as "peak-dose dyskinesia"), but about 5 percent of us experience dyskinesia when we have either too much or too little levodopa ("diphasic dyskinesia"). I am a good example of this: I develop symptoms whenever my medication isn't at the optimal level. In other words, I am among the unfortunate few who require tighter dosage control in order to avoid symptoms.

As Parkinson's progresses, most people need increasing doses of medication to control their symptoms. At higher doses, the risk of side effects and dyskinesia increases. At some point, the side effects of the medications become just as disabling as the Parkinson's symptoms themselves, leaving surgery as the final treatment option.

❚ Combination Drugs ❚

Stalevo is a combination of levodopa-carbidopa and enta-capone in a single pill. For some people, Stalevo extends the benefit of levodopa, allowing for improved control of Parkinson's symptoms. I have been on Stalevo for more than a year, and I find that it has reduced my off time.

❚ Other Drugs

In addition to dopamine agonists and levodopa-carbidopa, other drugs may be prescribed to make the levodopa more effective or to minimize side effects. These include the following:

❚ *COMT inhibitors.* Entacapone (Comtan) and tolcapone (Tasmar) are COMT inhibitors, which help to reduce the amount of off time in people already taking levodopa-carbidopa. (COMT stands for catecholamine-O-methyltransferase.) These drugs can allow the person with Parkinson's to take as much as 25 percent less levodopa, which helps to minimize the side effects. About 5 percent of entacapone users experience diarrhea; about 15 percent of tolcapone users experience severe diarrhea. People taking tolcapone should have their liver function tested on a regular basis as well. (The drugs can also cause the urine to turn a dark yellow-orange color, but this is not harmful.)

❚ *MAO-B inhibitors.* Selegiline (Eldepryl, Deprenyl, and Zelapar) are MAO-B inhibitors, which slow the breakdown of dopamine in the brain and help ease Parkinson's symptoms, especially in people in the early stages of the disease. (MAO-B stands for monoamine oxidase B, an enzyme in the body that degrades or breaks down levodopa in the brain.) These drugs can be used with levodopa-carbidopa to increase on time. Side effects of selegiline include insomnia, vivid dreams, hallucinations, and low blood pressure when standing. Side effects are more common in older people. People taking some types of antidepressants should not take selegiline.

In clinical trials, a new MAO-B inhibitor known as Azilect has been found to be effective as both a stand-alone drug and a levodopa enhancer. Azilect, taken once a day, helps control Parkinson's symptoms and may also slow progression of the disease. The drug has been approved for use in Canada, but it has not yet been approved for use in the United States.

❚ *Anticholinergics.* Trihexyphenidyl (Artane), benztropine mesylate (Cogentin) procyclidine (Kemadrin), and biperiden HCl (Akineton) are anticholinergics, which help reduce tremor and rigidity. They have been in use since the 1940s, but are no longer used widely because more efficient drugs have largely taken their place. Anticholinergics can produce significant side effects, especially in older people. These include memory loss, dry mouth, hallucinations, sleepiness, and constipation, among others.

❚ *Amantadine.* Amantadine, which is sold under the brand name Symmetrel, helps reduce dyskinesia. (Originally prescribed as an antiviral agent to treat the flu, it was also found to reduce the symptoms of Parkinson's disease.) In addition to reducing symptoms, amantadine may also offer some neuroprotective effect, protecting the existing dopamine cells from injury. Side effects include nausea, vomiting, hallucinations, insomnia, agitation, dry mouth, ankle swelling, and uneven, marbled purplish skin tone. For reasons not well understood, as many as one out of three people get no real benefit from amantadine, even though others experience a dramatic reduction in Parkinson's symptoms.

❚ *Botulinum toxin.* Botulinum toxin type A (Botox) and type B (Myobloc) have been used to treat some Parkinson's symptoms by interfering with how the muscles contract. The drugs have been somewhat helpful in treating foot dystonia (painful cramping of the foot) and excessive drooling. The benefit is temporary—two or three months—but the drug is considered very safe.

▌ Managing Dyskinesia

Dyskinesia is the medical term for irregular writhing and dancelike movements. Fast movements are called *chorea;* slow movements are called *athetosis;* very slow, virtually frozen posturing of the neck, trunk, and limbs is called *dystonia.*

Dyskinesia is not a symptom of PD, but a side effect of the levodopa-carbidopa used to treat the disease. Studies indicate that about one-third of Parkinson's patients develop dyskinesia four to six years after starting levodopa-carbidopa therapy, and almost 90 percent develop dyskinesia after nine years on the drug.

Treatment of dyskinesia typically involves adjusting the dosage of medication by lowering the dose of levodopa-carbidopa and adding a dopamine agonist or other medications, such as Symmetrel (amantadine) or a COMT inhibitor. If changes in medication aren't effective, a person with Parkinson's may need to consider surgery to minimize dependence on levodopa-carbidopa.

▌ The Future of a Parkinson's Patch ▌

Researchers have experimented with a once-daily transdermal patch for a new dopamine agonist known as rotigotine. The 85-week study involved 137 people with early-stage Parkinson's disease. The participants using the patch reported immediate improvement in their Parkinson's symptoms. Researchers theorize that the patch may be able to provide two to three years of control of Parkinson's symptoms.

Unlike oral medications, the patch provides a continuous dose of medicine. People don't need to worry about when to take their drugs. In the study the most common side effects were nausea, skin irritation at the patch site, dizziness, vomiting, and insomnia. The drug remains investigational, but it may be available in the next few years.

▌Using Medications Safely ▌

Here are some basic guidelines for using medications safely.

- Never stop taking any type of Parkinson's medication without discussing the matter with your doctor. Some Parkinson's medications need to be slowly tapered off rather than stopped cold turkey to avoid a worsening of symptoms.
- If you experience negative side effects—or if a medication does not appear to be useful—discuss the matter with your doctor. Do not change your dose without consulting your doctor.
- Always begin with the lowest possible dose and increase if necessary. Watch for side effects.
- If you experience side effects from levodopa-carbidopa treatment, ask your doctor about lowering the dose of the drug and adding a dopamine agonist.
- When changing a medication, allow two to four weeks

for your body to adjust before deciding whether it is having a beneficial effect. It can take several weeks for your system to adjust to the new medication or dosage.

- Stick to a regular medication schedule. Keeping a steady amount of medication in your system will help reduce the likelihood of motor fluctuations.
- Before taking any new medication, ask your physician and pharmacist to review all of the medications you are taking and note any possible drug interactions or combined side effects. Many people with Parkinson's take multiple drugs, increasing the likelihood of experiencing a dangerous interaction.

Some drug combinations should be avoided. For example:

- Antacid medications such as Tagamet, Zantac, and Pepcid should be taken two hours before or after levodopa-carbidopa to allow proper absorption of both medicines.
- Antipsychotic medications used to treat schizophrenia and mania can counteract the benefits of dopamine-stimulating drugs.
- Selegiline can interact with some antidepressants, causing a serotonergic crisis—high blood pressure, headache, high heart rate, chest pain, and high temperature.
- Antivomiting drugs can interfere with dopamine activity and worsen Parkinson's symptoms.
- Selegiline should never be given with Demerol (a painkiller often used after surgery) due to a risk of a change in heart rhythm.

▌ To Medicate or Not to Medicate?

Deciding what medication to take and when to start taking it can be quite difficult. You should develop a treatment plan with your doctor, although you should always be willing to reevaluate the plan and make adjustments as necessary. While you may hear about the importance of delaying medication until symptoms worsen, you should not compromise your daily life or live with symptoms you consider debilitating.

In the very early stages of the disease, you may not need medication at all. You may notice an occasional twitch or tremor that does not really interfere with your daily activities. When your motor function is impaired to the point that your Parkinson's symptoms interfere with your independence or your ability to do what you want to do, then you might consider using medication.

▌ Age Matters

The approach to treatment differs for younger and older people with Parkinson's. As a rule, people over 70 tend to skip the dopamine agonists and turn to levodopa-carbidopa as the first medication of choice. Often older people have trouble tolerating dopamine agonists without suffering side effects, including confusion and hallucinations.

In contrast, younger people often use dopamine agonists to manage their symptoms early in the disease, in part because younger people experience fewer side effects from these drugs than older people. In addition, younger people often have decades ahead of them to manage their Parkinson's symptoms, and many of the drugs will eventually lose their effectiveness, so many doctors try to delay the introduction of levodopa-carbidopa as long as possible. Most people with young-onset Parkinson's disease start out by using dopamine agonists, amantadine, and anticholinergics, adding levodopa-carbidopa to the mix within three to five years. In most cases, they continue to take the dopamine agonists along with the levodopa-carbidopa so that they can take the smallest possible dose of the latter.

Younger people sometimes want to increase their medication to the point that they appear virtually free of Parkinson's symptoms. Often people with YOPD have small children at home and important careers; they're at the peak of their productive lives and they don't want to slow down and surrender to the Parkinson's. While taking ever-increasing amounts of medication may be tempting, the higher the dose of medication, the greater the risk of side effects.

A young person who experiences disabling motor symptoms that cannot be well-controlled using medication may find surgery an appealing alternative. This is discussed in Chapter 5.

5

Surgery for Parkinson's Disease

For more than two years, 37-year-old Kellie couldn't get out of bed. Her muscles ached and would spasm so often that she was essentially paralyzed. She also had severe dystonia, episodes when her muscles would contract and cramp, rendering her entire body painfully twisted for hours at a time. "My muscles would turn to stone; my whole body was like a rock," she said. At least twice a month she had to seek help from the hospital emergency room where she would receive intravenous muscle relaxants for up to 24 hours before she could move.

Kellie needed help taking care of her three young children; she couldn't walk and rarely left the house. She decided to try deep brain stimulation (DBS), a surgical treatment for Parkinson's disease. DBS surgery involves inserting a thin wire into the brain; the wire is attached to a computerized pulse generator (similar to a heart pacemaker).

"I had no options," she said. "I knew I wouldn't be like before I had Parkinson's, but if I wanted half a life back, I knew I had to have surgery."

After more than six months of medical tests and psychological exams, Kellie underwent the six-and-a-half-hour procedure. "I was awake during the surgery," she said. "My head was in a halo so I couldn't move, but I could talk to the doctors. I knew they found the right spot in my brain when my tremors stopped. I looked up and saw my doctor smiling."

A week after the initial surgery to implant the electrodes, Kellie had a second procedure to attach wires that ran under her skin from her brain to a pacemaker-like device implanted in her chest. When the electrodes were activated, she was "turned on."

"There was an immediate change. All I wanted to do was go home and let my children see me walk," she said. "I wanted them to see that I could get up again."

Kellie accepts that the benefits of surgery may last only a few years. "No one can tell me how long it will work: two years? five years? I don't know. I can't live for tomorrow; I took what the doctors could give me. They offered me some of my life back, and I took it."

∎ Rediscovering Surgery

In the first half of the 20th century, doctors did not have any effective drugs to offer Parkinson's patients, so they turned to brain surgery as a last resort when symptoms were severe. In essence, surgeons relieved the patients' symptoms by destroying the sections of the brain thought to control the involuntary movement associated with PD.

As you might imagine, this crude surgery was risky and often ineffective. The mortality rate for these procedures stood at around 12 percent, and many more suffered permanent side effects, such as speech difficulty and vision problems.

The treatment of Parkinson's disease was revolutionized in 1967 when Dr. George Cotzias discovered levodopa, an oral medication used to treat Parkinson's patients. Not surprisingly, the number of surgical procedures plummeted, since the drug was much safer than surgery.

As was discussed in Chapter 4, the medications aren't without their flaws; over time, many people experience problems with wearing off, and some continue to suffer symptoms that the medications couldn't control. Some people need to take medication every hour or two, and worse yet, some of us develop dyskinesia as a side effect of the medication, making the cure worse than the disease.

But in the world of Parkinson's, nothing stays still for long. By the 1980s, researchers were developing new equipment and surgical techniques that have made Parkinson's surgery much safer. While medication remains the first line of treatment for new patients, I believe we are on the threshold of a new era of medicine that will include both better drugs and better procedures—and one day these new treatments will make Parkinson's a disease of the past. This chapter will review DBS, which has become the surgery of choice for most people with Parkinson's, as well as traditional brain lesioning procedures that have been in use for 50 years. It will also cover several experimental surgical procedures that offer promise to Parkinson's patients in the coming years.

■ An Overview of Surgery

A surgeon operating on the brain of a Parkinson's patient is like an electrician correcting a short in the wiring of your home. In a person with PD, there is a problem with the electrical pathway in the final circuit from the thalamus to the motor cortex in the brain. The neurosurgeon can fix this problem in one of two basic ways: by electrically stimulating the circuit (DBS) or by rewiring the circuit using a technique known as lesioning (cutting a small hole in the brain, creating what can be thought of as a minor stroke). Each procedure will be discussed in greater detail in the following text. Both types of surgery have been found to improve motor function in people with advanced PD or in those who no longer respond well to medication.

Deep Brain Stimulation

In the late 1990s, deep brain stimulation revolutionized the surgical treatment of Parkinson's disease. The surgery involves inserting a thin wire and electrodes into the brain, linking the wire to a remote battery, and stimulating the brain at a high frequency (100 to 180 hertz). The electrodes are positioned in the brain; the wires run under the skin along the skull and down the neck, eventually crossing over to a pacemaker-sized battery pack in the chest wall. All of the wires remain under the skin. The device can be programmed by holding a computer over the skin near the pulse generator. The procedure was approved by the U.S. Food and Drug Administration for the treatment of Parkinson's disease in 1997.

DBS will not reverse all symptoms. Rather, DBS is said to "turn back the clock" by five to seven years. In other words, it does not eliminate all Parkinson's symptoms, but rather it tends to improve symptoms to the level they were a half decade before. It's not a perfect fix, but it is a significant improvement for most people.

"The surgery didn't help with my speech or swallowing problems," said Jeremy, 31. "I still need extra water when I take my pills, and there are times I still have trouble with the words I need to find. But I'm much better, and it has reduced my medication by 60 percent."

The physical changes associated with DBS are determined by the positioning of the electrodes.

■ DBS of the subthalamic nucleus offers about an 80 percent reduction in tremor, as well as a 65 percent reduction in rigidity, a 51 percent reduction in bradykinesia, and an 80 to

90 percent reduction in dyskinesia. It can be done on one or both sides of the brain. After the surgery, many patients can reduce their daily dose of Parkinson's medications by 30 to 50 percent.

▌ DBS of the thalamus reduces tremor in about 92 percent of Parkinson's patients. Unfortunately, this type of DBS does not significantly improve rigidity and bradykinesia, making it an effective treatment only in people with tremor-predominant PD.

At this point there isn't enough long-term data to know how lasting the benefits of this surgery may be, but many people who have had DBS continue to experience benefits more than 10 years later. Remember, Parkinson's is a degenerative disease; your condition will continue to deteriorate even if you have surgery.

In most cases, DBS is performed when the patient is awake. Typically, a person does not take medication for at least a day before surgery, so that the doctors can accurately determine how the exact placement of the probes affects movement.

The mortality rate for DBS is extremely low; there has been only one reported death in North America associated with the procedure. Approximately 4 percent of patients experience non-life-threatening infections. About 2 percent of patients experience serious permanent side effects, including difficulty opening eyelids, weakness, and numbness; additional temporary complications include seizures, confusion, infection, facial numbness, and dyskinesia. In addition, the system requires maintenance; the electrodes must be programmed and tested on a regular basis, and the battery pack inserted under the skin in the chest wall must be changed every two to five years.

In some cases, the surgery must be repeated because the electrodes need to be repositioned or replaced. That's what happened to Kellie.

"The doctors don't know why, but my electrodes moved a bit," Kellie said. "I needed to have another surgery; my husband calls it a warranty job." At this point, Kellie reports that her left hand is twisted and she can't bend her fingers. Sometimes she feels her left side pulling and her toes curling under. "It's a glitch," she said, "the doctors will take care of it."

In early October 2006 Kellie's surgeons repositioned the two leads that had fallen out of position. In addition, they added two more leads in Kellie's brain. Having four leads will enhance the doctors' ability to fine-tune the frequencies in Kellie's system.

Michael and I visited Kellie a few weeks after the second surgery. She was a different person than we had seen before; she was smiling from ear to ear, active, and vibrant. She had no tremors and few signs of the debilitating dystonia that had plagued her before her DBS surgery. I watched with tears of joy when she picked up 2-year-old Noah and gave him a big bear hug.

Based on such anecdotes, it is my impression that the quality of DBS is much better than it used to be. I knew some people who had DBS as little as five years ago who spoke in a monotone after the surgery. They were often depressed and moved in a zombie-like fashion. I think the procedure has been improved; I don't see those symptoms anymore in patients who have undergone DBS surgery recently. Kellie had no trouble talking; in fact, her voice was more animated than it had been before surgery. Her movements were fluid and her energy level was incredible. Most of the people I know who have had the surgery have had good results; in some cases, you wouldn't know they had Parkinson's at all.

We are beginning the journey toward DBS for Michael. Michael has had PD for 11 years now, and he's at a point where his on time is short-lived and his off time grows more frequent. For several months we have been preparing ourselves and our families for this exciting procedure. After spending time with Kellie, Michael has become convinced that DBS surgery is the right next step for him.

Lesioning: Pallidotomy and Thalamotomy

Lesioning involves using a heat-sensitive probe to make a small hole in the brain that will alter motor function and relieve Parkinson's symptoms. No wires or electrodes are left behind after the procedure. *Pallidotomy* refers to a lesion in the globus pallidus; *thalamotomy* refers to a lesion in the thalamus. Lesioning is usually performed on only one side of the brain, the side opposite the symptoms. (The left side of the brain controls motor function on the right side of the body and vice versa.) As with DBS, lesioning procedures are typically performed when the patient is awake.

Pallidotomy is the most common lesioning surgery for Parkinson's disease; it has been available for more than 50 years. Studies indicate that the procedure can help relieve tremors, rigidity, and bradykinesia by 15 to 50 percent, and dyskinesia by as much as 80 to 90 percent. Pallidotomy does not help people with problems involving walking and balance. Some people experience a dramatic improvement after surgery, but the benefits wane in the weeks and months that follow; others maintain a benefit for five years after the procedure. Pallidotomy is most often recommended for people with Parkinson's symptoms that cannot be controlled with medication, as well as for those with disabling dyskinesia.

Thalamotomy can help reduce Parkinson's tremor and essential tremor by as much as 90 percent, but it does not significantly reduce rigidity or bradykinesia. For this reason, thalamotomy is typically used only on patients with tremor-predominant PD or severe essential tremor that does not respond to medication.

The mortality rate for both pallidotomy and thalamotomy is less than 1 percent, a vast improvement from the 12 percent fatality rate in the 1950s. Most fatalities are caused by brain hemorrhage. Other serious neurological complications include weakness or numbness on the opposite side of the body, partial vision loss, slurred speech, depression, difficulty swallowing, and seizures. About 11 percent of people who have pallidotomy experience at least partial vision loss. These symptoms can be permanent, although they sometimes improve over a period of months or years, similar to how a patient may recover from a stroke.

"I Live More Than the Average Person"

I was diagnosed with Parkinson's disease at age 35. I was on medication for eight years, then the dyskinesia from the Sinemet got so unbearable that I wouldn't go out. I became a hermit. In 2004, I found a neurosurgeon who could help me with deep brain stimulation.

The surgery was a total success, but there were times I thought I wasn't going to make it. One time during surgery the doctor started to drill into my skull while I was awake; another time I felt the doctor stapling me shut. Even with that, it was all worth it. After the surgery, my mother cried and thanked the doctor for giving her son back.

I've been blessed with a new life. When my medication doesn't work late at night, I have a tremor, but during the day, I have my life.

I don't fall like I did before surgery. There are grab bars in every room of my house, but I don't need them anymore. I was in a wheelchair before the surgery; now I don't even need a walker. I can go out to eat without people staring at me; people don't look at me and wonder what's wrong with me.

I thank God every day for my new life. I have accepted my place in this life; this disease has opened my eyes. I am doing things now I never dreamed I would be doing. I've learned to help people, to comfort other people with

Parkinson's, and that's just a wonderful feeling. I counsel other people who have Parkinson's and I answer all their questions.

I know the benefits of DBS won't last forever, so I try to live more than the average person. I live two days for every one. I get up early and talk to people. I go and do; I never just sit in the house. I volunteer and give of myself. When my time is over, that's what I want to be remembered as—someone who gave of himself.

Life is unbelievable now. You never know what's around the corner in this life. One thing I do know is that the time I have left is not going to be spent feeling sorry for myself.

— *Michael L., Tennessee*

■ The Future of Surgery

For 25 years, surgeons have experimented with tissue transplantation for PD. The process involves moving living tissue rich in dopamine into the brain of a Parkinson's patient. The tissue comes from human fetuses, pig fetuses, or other parts of the patient's brain. More than 200 people with Parkinson's disease have had the procedure, with widely varying results. To date, these procedures have not been very successful; the approach is considered very experimental.

One of the most recent studies involving the procedure had to be stopped owing to the unacceptably high rate of disabling dyskinesia that occurred in patients who had the transplants. In fact, some of these patients required a pallidotomy to improve the dyskinesia that resulted from the tissue transplantation surgery.

I believe that stem-cell research and gene-therapy surgery will provide unimagined benefits to people with Parkinson's in the decades to come. At this point, these procedures are not available, but I remain optimistic that regenerative medicine will be the new frontier of the 21st century. (For more about gene therapy, stem cells, and the future of Parkinson's, see Chapter 17.)

"I'll Never Have DBS"

I've thoroughly researched surgery, and my doctors said I'm a good candidate, but I'll never have DBS. For me, I can't stand the side effects, especially the voice. A good 80 percent of the people I know who have had the surgery have found that it affects their voice. The area of the brain where they put the probes is near the areas that control speech. For some, their voices become nasal, like that of a deaf person, and they can't enunciate their words clearly. My voice already gets soft from the Parkinson's, but I don't want to lose the ability to sing.

Of the people I know who have had the operation, there's about a 60-40 chance that it will work well, without side effects. The odds aren't high enough for me. When it goes bad, it goes very bad.

Last, but certainly not least, it's a Band-Aid. It gives you five to seven years of better function. I don't want a Band-Aid—I want a cure.

Other friends tell me, "You will know when you're ready for surgery." I know they're telling me that the time will come when my life is so compromised that it will be worth the risk. I still have more good days than bad. I can walk. I can drive. I lead a relatively normal life. There are times when I have a bad two or three days in a row, but in general, I'm doing quite well.

— James, Texas

▌ Should You Have Surgery?

Most people with Parkinson's may not need surgery. At this point, my medications are working well enough that I don't think I need it—although I am very open to the idea if and when my situation changes. Deciding on surgery is a personal decision; no one can make it for you.

Surgery is typically done on people who are relatively young and in good overall health, who have severe symptoms or disabling dyskinesia that don't respond to medication. Some experts estimate that about 15 to 20 percent of people with PD could benefit from surgery. Initially, doctors withheld DBS until a patient could no longer tolerate medications for Parkinson's. In recent years, however, doctors have begun to recommend surgery for people earlier in the course of the disease to enhance quality of life.

Don't think of surgery as an alternative to medication. In a successful procedure, your symptoms will improve, but you will likely continue to need some medication. Prospective surgery patients must be carefully screened for preexisting psychiatric problems because the procedure has been known to worsen—in most cases temporarily—depression, anxiety, drug addiction, and other psychiatric problems.

Be sure you've worked with the best neurologist you can find to get the most you can from the medications out there before turning to an invasive surgery to ease your symptoms.

In recent years, DBS has become the procedure of choice among most neurologists, but the decision of which type of surgery you should have should be made by you and your neurologist together. More studies need to be done comparing DBS and lesioning, but most experts believe DBS has less risk of serious side effects. Lesioning is a one-time procedure—and any bad results can last a lifetime; DBS can be fine-tuned to some degree after the surgery.

But DBS isn't right for everyone. People who don't live near a facility that can maintain the DBS device, those who feel squeamish about having electrodes in their brain, those who don't want to have to maintain the battery pack, and those who need to take blood thinner may not be good candidates for DBS.

Be sure the neurosurgeon you work with has experience performing the procedure you choose and that the hospital where the surgery will be done has the latest equipment. Don't rush to the operating table; take time to get a second or third opinion. Learn everything you can about the procedure and talk to other people who have had it done. (Ask for referrals from your physician and reach out to people online and in support groups who can share their experiences with you.) You want to know everything you can before making such an important decision.

The following chapter looks at finding the right doctor. It is important to find a good doctor to work with you in managing the day-to-day challenges of living with Parkinson's, but it is absolutely essential to carefully select a neurosurgeon if you are considering surgery to deal with your Parkinson's.

6

Finding the Right Doctor

Finding the right doctor to help you with your Parkinson's can be exhausting. My friend, Karen, who was diagnosed with PD when she was 42 years old, had to virtually diagnose herself.

In the summer of 1998, Karen felt weak on her left side. She walked with an awkward gait because she couldn't lift the toes on her left foot when she walked; she couldn't wash her hair satisfactorily because she couldn't scrub her scalp with her left hand. She worried that she might have suffered a small stroke, but her family doctor performed various tests and insisted that everything was normal.

She went to a neurologist; he told her she was stressed and needed rest. He implied her symptoms were psychosomatic. She found another neurologist; he told her she was too young to have PD.

She turned to her computer and began to search for a diagnosis. "I went home and went online," Karen R. said. "I put 'Parkinson's disease' in the browser. The first website listed the symptoms; I had almost every one. I knew that was it. I wanted to know what I had, but I didn't want it to be Parkinson's disease. I wanted something curable. I wanted something temporary."

Karen R. made an appointment with another neurologist, but he could not see her for several weeks. In the meantime, she and her husband tuned in to a television special on ABC's *20/20* in which actor Michael J. Fox discussed his Parkinson's disease. "When he described his symptoms, he was speaking about me," Karen said. "I started to cry. My husband said, 'Stop—don't try to diagnose yourself.' But I knew. I just knew."

Eventually, Karen's doctor confirmed what she had feared for months: she had PD. "It may sound crazy, but I was glad to finally know what I was dealing with."

Like Karen R., most people with Parkinson's disease, especially young-onset Parkinson's, have a horror story to tell about finding the right doctor and getting the correct diagnosis. I would imagine that on average people with YOPD see three to five neurologists before finding one they like who is familiar with PD. Too often the people I meet tell me that their neurologists ruled out Parkinson's because they were too young or they didn't have all of the traditional symptoms. In this chapter, I hope to save you some time and trouble by helping you find a doctor who will be familiar with your condition and sensitive to your needs.

▌ Let the Search Begin

Whether you are trying to confirm a diagnosis of Parkinson's disease or need to work with a doctor to manage your condition, it is essential that you find a doctor you feel comfortable with and trust. If you have any questions about your diagnosis, be sure to seek a second opinion. A good doctor will respect your desire to learn as much as you can about your condition rather than feeling threatened by your decision to speak with another physician.

Don't be afraid of telling a doctor, "You're fired!" You want a doctor who will be your advocate and who will care about you. If you have any reservations about the doctor you're seeing, it's time to find another doctor.

You will want to establish a team of caregivers, possibly including:

▌ A general practitioner, who will address your overall health care

▌ A neurologist, who will manage your Parkinson's disease

▌ A movement-disorders specialist if your neurologist doesn't have experience in this field

▌ A physical therapist, who will help you develop an exercise program and find ways of meeting your specific physical challenges

▌ An expert on complementary or natural medicine, who will be able to recommend nutritional supplements, diet plans, herbs, exercise, and other parts of a balanced health regimen that may not be covered by a traditional physician

▌ A good pharmacist, one who is willing to answer your questions and knows about possible drug interactions

With all of your health-care providers—but especially your neurologist—look for someone with experience treating Parkinson's patients. While we would all prefer to be seen regularly by a seasoned movement-disorders specialist who is familiar with the latest research on PD, that is not always possible. I have both a local neurologist, whom I see every six weeks or so, and a movement-disorders specialist, whom I see two or three times a year. (It's a blessing that I don't need to see the movement-disorders specialist more often since his office is two hours from my home.)

There is an adage in the Parkinson's community: "When you've seen one Parkinson's patient, you've seen one Parkinson's patient." That's because each of us presents a unique combination of symptoms and sensitivities: we respond to medications differently, our symptoms progress at different speeds, we expect different levels of performance from our bodies. A doctor with experience treating a number of Parkinson's patients stands a better chance of understanding what *you* are going through and how he or she can help you. Early in the course of your illness, you should expect to see your neurologist every six to eight weeks. If a neurologist hands you a prescription and says, "See me in four months," find another neurologist. I still see my neurologist every six weeks, and I have had Parkinson's for almost seven years; I wouldn't have it any other way.

Start your search by collecting names of physicians in your area. Ask friends and relatives for suggestions. You might also contact a local or regional Parkinson's center and ask for a referral. You may want to check the "Physician Select" service at the American Medical Association's website: www.ama-assn.org. This site can give you lists of doctors by specialty who practice in your area.

Another option is the website run by the Administrators in Medicine, a group of state medical board directors, at www.docboard.org/docfinder.html. This site includes physician lists from the American Board of Medical Specialties, state medical and osteopathic boards of directors, and the National Board of Medical Examiners, among others.

Many health insurance plans can provide lists of specialists who participate in your plan. Check your policy to determine whether you will need to restrict your search to doctors on an approved list.

Before choosing a physician, set up an interview or an initial appointment to assess how you feel about the doctor. Because Parkinson's medications need to be adjusted with some regularity, you will develop an ongoing relationship with your neurologist, so you want to be sure you find someone you like.

∎ Ask Questions

Never be afraid to ask questions. I recommend that you write them down and bring them with you. It's all too easy to be sidetracked in conversation or be hurried along and not remember to ask every question if you don't take the time to write them down ahead of time.

Here are a few questions you could consider asking.

About Parkinson's Disease

▋ Do you have expertise working with Parkinson's patients?

▋ How many Parkinson's patients do you see?

▋ How many people with young-onset Parkinson's do you see?

▋ How often do you see your Parkinson's patients?

▋ What is your opinion about surgery for Parkinson's?

▋ What is your success rate using surgery?

▋ What is your opinion about complementary or alternative medicine? What about the use of nutrition and nutritional supplements in the treatment of Parkinson's disease?

▋ May I have the names of several patients with Parkinson's disease who would be willing to speak with me as references?

Practical Matters

▋ Are you accepting new patients?

▋ Do you accept my insurance plan?

▋ Do you accept Medicare?

▋ What are your customary fees?

▋ At which hospitals do you have staff privileges?

▋ How long does it usually take to get a routine appointment?

▋ Do you set aside time every day for emergency appointments?

▋ Does your practice have a telephone query line?

▋ Do you answer questions sent by e-mail?

▋ Do you have evening or weekend hours?

About the Practice

■ Do you practice alone or are you part of a group?
■ Who covers for you if I have a problem while you are out of town or unavailable?
■ Are there any fees if I need to cancel an appointment?
■ Are you certified by a medical specialty board? (For more information on certification, see "Checking Out Your Doctor.")

Ask Yourself

■ Were the doctor and staff courteous?
■ Did I have to wait long?
■ Did I get all of my questions answered?
■ Did I feel rushed?
■ Is the location of the office convenient?
■ Would I feel more comfortable with a doctor who was younger? older?

■ Checking Out Your Doctor ■

You may want to check out your doctor before you schedule an appointment. With a few clicks of the computer mouse or a couple of phone calls, you can make sure that your doctor is a member in good standing with a medical board of certification and you can see if he or she has been the target of any disciplinary actions.

Specialty medical certification is a sign that your doctor has gone above and beyond to develop—and demonstrate—expertise in a given field of study, such as neurology or surgery. In most cases, specialty certification requires several years of additional training; in addition, the physician must pass a proficiency exam. Board certification offers some external measure of a doctor's knowledge, but it is certainly possible to receive good care from a doctor who is not board-certified.

The American Board of Medical Specialties (ABMS) is a private organization that certifies specialty boards. You can call toll-free at 800-776–2378 to find out if a physician's certifying board is ABMS-approved. The ABMS can also give you the phone number of the certifying specialty board so that you can verify that the physician is actually certified. You can also check the website at www.certifieddoctor.org.

To find out if disciplinary actions have been filed against a particular doctor, contact Public Citizen at 202-588-1000, or do a search at their website, www.citizen.org, for articles on "Questionable Doctors."

▌ Making the Most of Your Appointment

Like the squeaky sound your car makes every day, except when you visit your mechanic, Parkinson's symptoms can be hard to pin down. You may have a symptom that annoys you for weeks, but it suddenly disappears on the day you have an appointment with the neurologist. Since your PD symptoms can turn on and off without notice, you can make the most of your doctor's visit by bringing a log or journal listing the frequency of symptoms and the dose of medication you are taking. This log can be helpful for both you and your doctor in keeping track of how you are responding to medication. (See Appendix for sample logs.)

Here are a few more ideas that can help you use your time—and the doctor's—more efficiently.

▌ If you are a new patient, ask the doctor to mail or fax the information forms to you in advance. Filling out the tiny boxes on health forms can be particularly trying for someone with Parkinson's disease, who may write slowly or illegibly.

▌ Bring a spouse, friend, relative, or another caregiver with you to your appointments. This person can take notes during the appointment and help clarify any instructions if the advice you receive is not clear when you get home.

▌ Always tell your doctor about your most pressing concerns at the beginning of your appointment. Don't wait for the doctor to ask you questions. Your appointment time may be limited and you want to cover the most important issues first.

▌ Always bring written records of *all* the medications you are taking, including over-the-counter drugs.

▌ Always tell your doctor if you are taking any vitamins, herbs, or other treatments for your Parkinson's disease or any other medical problem. Your doctor needs a complete picture of everything that is going on inside your body.

▌ Tell your doctor everything—even the embarrassing symptoms that you would rather keep to yourself. If you're having a problem with incontinence or impotence or falling, your doctor needs to know. You can only get help for your symptoms if the doctor knows you are having them.

▌ If your doctor has performed any tests, call the office if you don't hear the results within a couple of days. Even the most well-intentioned doctors can neglect to keep you informed of results if you don't ask.

While finding a good doctor is an essential step in managing your PD, you will also benefit from learning the essentials of alternative medicine and self-care. The following section looks at exercise, diet, attitude, and rest, as well as the importance of treating depression and learning to take advantage of support groups.

PART THREE

Alternative Medicine and Self-Care

7

Exercise:
The Importance of Movement

"I've had Parkinson's disease for eleven years, but it isn't any more than a nuisance in my life," said David, age 70. "I think one of the secrets of my being so free of symptoms is that I walk five miles every day. It takes discipline, but I've made a commitment to it."

David had been a runner for 25 years, and his doctors have suggested that his excellent overall health has helped limit his PD symptoms. "My symptoms have increased and I have a tremor in my right hand, so I drink from my left hand," he said. "I've been able to not let the disease change my life."

Every morning, David and his wife exercise together. "It's been terrific for our marriage," he said. "I might not be as disciplined about exercising if I didn't have the incentive of having Parkinson's, but I know the walking helps control the disease. I may get worse even if I exercise, but so far I'm doing fine and today is a great day."

Like David, most people with Parkinson's disease know how important it is to exercise. But let's be honest: if you're like me, there are days you feel lethargic and exhausted from the moment you roll out of bed. On those mornings, just putting my feet on the floor hurts, and the thought of pushing myself through an exercise routine seems overwhelming. Some days I convince myself to get moving and see if the pain and stiffness wear off; other days I give myself permission to rest and take the day off.

Life with Parkinson's is like that: unpredictable. I honestly can't tell why some days are easy and others are more difficult, but I know that my life is less stressful when I accept my feelings for the day rather than trying to control them. I cannot push the Parkinson's into remission by force of will; if I could, I would have been cured years ago! Instead, I find my life is smoother when I adapt my expectations based on how active my symptoms are at any given moment of any given day.

When it comes to exercise, I try to work out at least three to four times a week, and most of the time I am able to meet my goal. I don't think it has anything to do with my Parkinson's, but I find that the more I exercise, the more I want to exercise. (And, conversely, the more I slack off, the more I want to slack off.) Exercise is a habit, and if you do it regularly, your body starts to expect it.

Research indicates that there are several forms of muscle weakness involved with Parkinson's, including weakening of the pulmonary muscles. While you may find that you are not able to bench-press as much as you did in the past, the important thing is that you are doing something to help build strength. We understand that the Parkinson's may make it more challenging to perform certain exercises on certain days, but everyone needs to exercise, especially people with Parkinson's.

■ The Benefits of Exercise

Exercise offers significant health benefits, whether or not you have Parkinson's disease. It improves your physical and emotional health, reduces your risk of serious illness, increases your energy level, and provides a social outlet. For people with Parkinson's, regular exercise can help improve flexibility, reduce muscle stiffness, and slow the advancement of Parkinson's symptoms.

James, 51, feels better if he exercises daily. "I play disc golf—Frisbee golf," he said. "I play thirty-six holes a day. The course is near my house, and it's two and a half miles long. Instead of putting a ball into a hole, you throw the disc into the basket. It's had a great benefit for my Parkinson's.

"The first time I played I could barely lift my arms and complete nine holes, but I kept at it," James said. "It took nine months before I could complete an eighteen-hole course. It's a little bit hobby and a little bit compulsion."

I find that exercise can create a momentum that carries me through the day. It improves both my physical state and my state of mind. A number of studies back me up on this. For example, a study published in 2006 in the journal *Movement Disorders* reported that people with Parkinson's disease who participated in a combined aerobic and strength-training program showed significant improvements in their quality of life, including emotional, social, and physical measures. Other studies have shown that people with Parkinson's disease who exercise regularly feel more independent and have a higher quality of life.

"Parkinson's disease is like a vine," said Karen R., 56. "If you sit still, it will grow all over you and slow you down. You need to keep moving." That's not to say that you can keep your PD on hold by grabbing your running shoes or swimsuit and heading for the gym or pool. You'll need to work with your doctor to develop an exercise program that works for you. But remember, it's never too late to start an exercise program. While I was active before I received my diagnosis, I didn't follow a regular exercise regime. Now I know that I tend to feel better on the days I make time for exercise, so I try to make it a priority every day. It is important to remember the old adage "Move it or lose it"; the more we move, the longer we will keep moving.

Note: Always check with your doctor before beginning an exercise program. Your doctor may be able to point out specific exercises that may be helpful—or potentially harmful—to you.

■ Working Up a Workout Plan

A well-rounded exercise program includes three components: aerobic fitness, muscle strength, and flexibility. I'm not suggesting that you spend hours flexing in the gym or sweating to the oldies in aerobic dance classes, but you should try to include all three types of exercise in your program. It's easier than you may think.

For some people, it can be as simple as walking the dog. "I try to walk with my dog several times a day," said Carol, 63. "He's a little Chihuahua. I walk a quarter of a mile. I am afraid of falling, so I use a walker. It's good to get out and get moving every day."

Tom, 67, continues to lift weights, stretch, and work out on a treadmill despite his Parkinson's disease.

I find exercise very uplifting, and I believe it is very important to the Parkinson's patient. Exercise has always been an important part of my life. I always exercised, and I was afraid that I was going to be told the exercise was going to be bad for me now. I did some research and found that people who exercise do better with their Parkinson's.

I read about a man in Los Angeles who has run thirteen marathons with Parkinson's. It's easy for people to be deceived and think that all they can do is sit around and watch television. You need a proactive mind-set; you need to do things purposefully to treat the Parkinson's. You need to schedule your exercise—and rest—to make good habits a part of your daily routine.

Aerobic Fitness

The word *aerobic* means "using oxygen." During aerobic exercise, your heart and lungs work harder than normal to provide your muscles with the oxygen they demand, and you breathe heavily and steadily to meet your body's increased need for oxygen. During anaerobic exercise, your heart and lungs cannot meet your body's increased need for oxygen for longer than a minute or two, and you are left gasping and wheezing for breath (even if you're in good shape). Jogging around the block is aerobic exercise. Sprinting to catch the bus is anaerobic exercise.

Some people with Parkinson's may laugh at the thought of either jogging or sprinting. I understand; I tend to freeze when I start running. But you can find a form of aerobic exercise that can work for you. I enjoy lap swimming, which is easy on the joints. It hasn't happened to me yet, but I am aware of the risk of freezing in the water, so I swim half-laps; I go back and forth across the shallow end of the pool so I can stand if I need to. I sometimes lose my balance during exercise, and I find it easier to be in the water so I can catch myself if I start to fall.

Studies have found that aerobic exercise not only helps people with Parkinson's disease improve their aerobic capacity, but it also helps with movement problems, such as freezing. A 16-week study of the impact of aerobic exercise on people with Parkinson's, published in *NeuroRehabilitation* in 2002, found that participants experienced significant improvement in aerobic capacity and improved their ability to initiate and perform appropriate movements.

So what do you need to do to enjoy the marvelous benefits of aerobic conditioning? First, choose an activity that involves the rhythmic, repeated use of the major muscle groups, such as walking, swimming, yoga, or tai chi. When done regularly—three times a week for at least 20 to 30 minutes—aerobic activities improve the efficiency of the heart, lungs, and muscles.

For maximum benefit, you need to work hard enough—but not too hard. Your pulse rate (number of heartbeats per minute) is your body's speedometer: it tells you how fast your heart is going and if you need to speed up or slow things down to exercise in your optimal conditioning zone. Cardiovascular conditioning takes place when your heart beats at 70 to 85 percent of its maximum safe rate. You maximum heart rate is approximately 220 minus your age.

Consider turning on some music before starting your workout. A study published in 2000 in the journal *Psychosomatic Medicine* found that people with Parkinson's disease who participated in music therapy—including rhythmic and free body movement to music—experienced significant reduction in bradykinesia (slowness of movement) and rigidity.

In addition to your regular formal workout, make an effort to remain active. Michael doesn't follow a designated exercise regimen, but he is very active every day, chopping down trees, building ramps, and rebuilding cars. He also takes walks and goes fishing, which can provide some exercise if the fish are biting. His balance is very good and he gets a lot of satisfaction out of doing things for himself. He also enjoys showing off that his balance is better than mine. This usually leads to some good challenges that are not only fun, but get us moving.

Don't forget the importance of play. Every once in a while, I join Michael and the kids in a game of tackle football. I've tackled them, they've tackled me, and, frankly, there have been times I've tackled myself by freezing and falling on my face! That's part of living with Parkinson's disease. And when I fall down and eat a mouthful of grass, I try to take it all in stride as part of the game.

Another game that is one of my favorites is "Let's see who will get pushed into the pool first." Even though Michael has better balance than I do, I sometimes manage to get the upper hand and he ends up taking a dive into the pool. Living in Florida provides us with several ways to keep active. We like to splash around in the Gulf of Mexico or walk on the beach and collect shells and end the day strolling down the beach to catch the glorious sunsets that take your breath away.

The important thing to remember is that getting moving does not have to mean drudgery and it can come in many forms. In fact, the more joy you get from the activity, the more positive effects it will have on your body and mental outlook.

Muscle Strength

There's only one way to prevent muscle weakness and atrophy—exercise. Muscle weakness is not an inevitable side effect of Parkinson's disease, and it is not a side effect of aging. You can keep your muscles strong and supple by performing strength-building exercises, such as weight lifting and isometric exercises.

As an added benefit for people with Parkinson's, strength training helps stabilize the joints and reduce the risk of falls and injury. Researchers have also found that strength training helps people with Parkinson's disease improve their walking velocity and stride length. A 2001 article published in the *American Journal of Physical Medicine and Rehabilitation* found that people with Parkinson's disease who participated in an eight-week program of resistance training twice a week experienced significant improvements in their stride length, walking velocity, and posture. Since most people with Parkinson's have some trouble with gait and movement at least some of the time, it's clear that some type of strength training should be part of your exercise program.

Another study compared two groups of people with Parkinson's disease—one group participated in a 10-week program of strength training and balance exercises and the other did not exercise at all. The exercise group experienced significant improvement in balance, as well as some improvement in knee flexibility and strength. The couch-potato group showed no improvement in balance and a significant reduction in strength.

Without strength training, you will lose muscle mass and strength. The average American loses 10 to 20 percent of muscle strength between the ages of 20 and 50, and then another 25 to 30 percent between 50 and 70. Fortunately, you're never too old to grow stronger. One study found that 90-year-old nursing-home residents increased their muscle strength by up to 180 percent in an eight-week weight-lifting program.

Designing a weight-training program is beyond the scope of what we can cover in this book. I recommend that you get a list of recommended exercises from your doctor or from a physical therapist with experience working with people with Parkinson's disease. Information from Parkinson's organizations or books and exercise videos may also be helpful.

▮ A Workout Just for You ▮

Several national Parkinson's disease organizations offer materials about exercise:

- "Parkinson's Disease: Fitness Counts" is a free manual from the National Parkinson Foundation; 1501 NW Ninth Avenue, Miami, FL 33136; 800-327-4545.
- "Home Exercise Program for Patients with Parkinson's Disease" is available free from the American Parkinson Disease Association, 1250 Hylan Blvd., Suite 4B, Staten Island, NY 10305; 800-223-2732; www.apdaparkinson. com.
- "Exercises for the Parkinson's Patient, with Hints for Daily Living" is available from the Parkinson's Disease Foundation, 1359 Broadway, Suite 1509, New York, NY 10018; 212-923-4700; www.pdf.org.
- Motivating Moves offers videos and DVDs with seated

and standing exercise programs designed specifically for people with Parkinson's. To order a video or DVD or for more information, visit their website, www.motivating-moves.com.

Flexibility

Flexibility is the polar opposite of rigidity, one of the defining symptoms of Parkinson's disease. Flexibility involves more than touching your toes; it involves maintaining the range of motion in your joints, which can allow you to perform your everyday activities without discomfort. Maintaining flexibility makes you less prone to muscle strains and sprains, and it helps support your joints. At our support group at church, we sometimes take a few minutes to form a big circle and do some stretching and range-of-motion exercises before we work on stretching our faith.

Stretching is the key to preserving your flexibility. Start with 10-minute stretching sessions in the morning and evening and work you way toward 20-minute sessions twice a day. You'll want to move and stretch your entire body—neck, shoulders, waist; fingers, wrists, elbows, arms; toes, ankles, legs, and hips—through their full range of motion in every direction. Gently stretch and hold, then repeat two or three times. Never bounce or force yourself to stretch to the point of discomfort. Your Parkinson's disease has already made your muscles stiff, and you don't want to injure them by over-stretching.

Stretch your face by opening your jaw, raising your eyebrows, smiling wide, blinking your eyes, sticking out your tongue, and making exaggerated facial expressions. End with a gentle face massage. Parkinson's disease affects even the tiny muscles in your face; these muscles need a workout, too.

Again, a specific list of stretches is more than we can cover here, so talk to your doctor or physical therapist about a full-body stretching plan. Many programs for people with Parkinson's can be done while sitting in a chair or lying in bed first thing in the morning.

▮ Getting Started

Don't try to be a hero and do too much, too soon. Start your exercise program slowly, and gradually increase the frequency and intensity of activity. Parkinson's disease may make your workouts a little slower than you might like, and you might need to think about each step or each movement rather than taking it all for granted. That's okay—each exercise step you take is a step in the direction of better health. Don't worry about how fast you move. You'll reach your goal; it just may take a little bit longer than it would for someone else.

You need to make a commitment to exercise every day that you can. If you miss a few days of exercise, don't feel guilty and throw in the towel (literally). Instead, just get back into it.

Of course, never perform any exercise that causes pain. You don't want to pull a muscle or irritate a joint. If you're feeling off balance, sit down until you're more settled. The last thing you want to do is risk injury or a fall. Tomorrow is another day, and, as anyone with Parkinson's disease knows, symptoms can vary widely from one day to the next.

▮ Grab a Partner

When performing certain exercises—such as swimming, hiking, sailing, or other potentially dangerous activities—don't work out alone. You need to acknowledge that Parkinson's disease increases your risk of losing your balance and falling, or freezing and having trouble in the water. Even if you haven't had problems in the past, you cannot anticipate when some new Parkinson's symptom will rear its ugly head. In other words, just because you haven't had a problem with freezing or falling, it doesn't mean you won't the next time you go out to exercise. This doesn't mean that you should stay home; it means that you should always exercise with a friend or family member who can keep an eye on you if you need help for any reason.

If you do exercise alone, always carry a cell phone and let someone know where you are going, when you are leaving, and when you will return. (Of course, that's good advice if you don't have Parkinson's disease, too.)

Another excellent option is to join an exercise group at a local community center, YMCA, or medical clinic. Some facilities offer classes designed for people with Parkinson's disease. If you enroll in a regular exercise class, tell the instructor about your Parkinson's before the start of the class. You may want to contact your local Parkinson's organization, if you have one, to see if exercise classes may be available. Our local organization, Parkinson's Association of Southwest Florida, has an extensive list of locations and classes, including stretching and exercises, speech classes, and water exercise programs. These classes are free to people with PD.

In addition to your exercise plan, you can use diet and nutritional supplements to minimize your Parkinson's symptoms. This is discussed in Chapter 8.

8

Nourish Yourself: The Importance of Diet and Nutritional Supplements

By the time Doris had had Parkinson's disease for 15 years, she needed help with almost all of her daily activities. She was only in her midfifties but she couldn't walk from the bathroom to the bed without assistance; she couldn't dress herself or prepare her meals. Everything changed when she read that changing her diet and taking nutritional supplements could prevent her symptoms.

At that point in her life, Doris felt she had nothing to lose by changing her lifestyle:

I ate food rich in the amino acid GABA (gamma-amino-butyric acid) and I took a slew of supplements—B vitamins, GABA, alpha-lipoic acid, and lots of others. I took the supplements for about three months, but I saw results very quickly. Within a few weeks, I almost felt normal. As I got better, I was able to exercise again. When I started, I couldn't swing my arms when I walked, if I could walk at all. When my motor skills came back to me, I started walking, biking, playing racquetball, and working out with weights at the gym. I got my health back.

I remember sitting in my support group and seeing the other people who were struggling, and I felt completely normal. It's obvious that for me nutrition is very important. The better I followed the program, the better I felt. I've proven that for myself.

I stayed with it for about a year, but I reached the point that I felt so normal that I got away from my good habits. I got a little cocky, I think. I felt so good that I thought I could eat some key lime pie here, some pizza there. Before long I was eating the same nonnutritious foods I had been, and I gave up on the supplements. It doesn't make any sense that I went off the program when I started to feel good, but that's what happened—and then my Parkinson's came back.

I went back on the diet and supplements and I felt better within two weeks. I think I've learned my lesson—I hope I've learned my lesson.

While I haven't had the disease-transforming experience that Doris had, I do believe nutritional supplements and diet can strengthen the body and minimize Parkinson's symptoms. I take a handful of supplements every day, but frankly, I cannot afford to pay for a wide range of over-the-counter products as well as our prescription medications. (Some supplements are available by prescription—and covered by insurance—but the cost of the vast majority will not be reimbursed.)

In my experience, most doctors dismiss nutrition and supplements as unimportant. I believe that each of us should do all we can to confront our Parkinson's with every tool we have. If adding certain foods to our diets or nutrients to our list of daily vitamins helps control our PD, we should definitely be open to trying it. Clearly, there are serious limitations to the prescription medications available for PD; if natural therapies work, I completely support their use.

While there is a wide range of nutritional supplements that may strengthen your overall health, this chapter will focus on the supplements most likely to provide therapeutic benefits. There are, of course, many others. I encourage you to learn about them and develop a program that best addresses the deficiencies in your personal situation.

One word of caution: be sure to tell your doctor about any supplements you take or special changes you make to your diet. At least 40 percent of PD patients use some alternative therapies—including vitamins, herbs, massage, and acupuncture—but more than half do not tell their physicians about these treatments. In some cases, there can be drug interactions or side effects from nonprescription medications.

▌ Antioxidants

Oxygen is essential to life, but oxygen can be damaging when it is at the wrong place at the wrong time. As oxygen travels through the body, many molecules it encounters lose an electron, making them chemically unstable. These ions or free radicals are highly reactive, and they eventually steal an electron from another molecule, leaving that molecule damaged. This oxidative damage may play a role in the formation of Parkinson's disease, as well as other chronic illnesses.

The brain consumes about 20 percent of the oxygen in the body, and with that high level of oxygen consumption evidence shows an increase in the number of free radicals in the brain. The problem becomes worse when the number of free radicals is further increased by the toxic burden of household chemicals, pesticides, and other toxic exposures.

Antioxidants—whether consumed as food or nutritional supplements—can help the body fight free-radical damage and stabilize the reactive oxygen molecules by freely donating extra electrons. Antioxidants include vitamin C, vitamin E, and selenium, among others.

Vitamin C

One-fourth of all Americans do not get even the minimum amount of vitamin C—60 milligrams—that cells need to perform basic biological functions. In the body, vitamin C (ascorbic acid) helps with tissue and collagen growth, wound healing, adrenal gland function, and healthy gums, in addition to serving as a powerful antioxidant. Studies have found plasma levels of vitamin C to be significantly lower in people with Parkinson's disease, compared to healthy controls.

Dosage: Take 2,000 milligrams of vitamin C daily in divided doses (half in the morning, half at night), or follow package directions.

Vitamin E

Vitamin E helps improve circulation, promotes healthy blood clotting, lowers blood pressure, helps prevent cataracts, and repairs damaged tissue. It may also play a role in preventing cancer and cardiovascular disease. Studies have found the risk of PD significantly reduced among men and women who consumed moderate levels of vitamin E from food, rather than supplements.

PD patients who have high blood pressure or who are on an anticoagulant (blood thinner) such as Coumadin (warfarin) should not take vitamin E supplements without a doctor's approval.

Dosage: Take 400 IU of vitamin E daily, or follow package directions.

Selenium

Selenium is a powerful antioxidant, especially when combined with vitamin E. In the body, this trace element helps form the antioxidant selenium-glutathione peroxidase. It is also needed for pancreatic function, tissue elasticity, and red blood cell metabolism.

Studies have shown that people with chronic illnesses such as Parkinson's disease may have low levels of selenium. For best results, take selenomethionine, rather than sodium selenite or sodium selenate.

Dosage: Take 100 micrograms of selenium daily, or follow product directions.

▌Coenzyme Q10

Coenzyme Q10—also known as ubiquinone and CoQ10—allows the cells to produce energy. CoQ10 acts as an antioxidant by binding to toxic free radicals, preventing them from killing healthy cells. Research has shown that people with Parkinson's disease tend to be deficient in CoQ10.

Results of the first placebo-controlled, multicenter clinical trial of CoQ10 suggest that it can slow disease progression in patients with early-stage PD. Researchers at the University of California, San Diego, believe that CoQ10 works by improving the function of mitochondria.

The researchers found that taking CoQ10 was well tolerated and significantly increased the level of CoQ10 in the blood. Compared to those not receiving the supplement, study participants receiving 1,200 milligrams of CoQ10 daily had 44 percent less decline in mental function, motor function, and ability to carry out activities of daily living, such as feeding or dressing themselves. Other participants who received either 300 or 600 milligrams of CoQ10 developed slightly less disability than the placebo group, but the effects were less than those in the group that received the highest dose. Additional research on the neuroprotective capabilities of CoQ10 is currently being conducted by the Department of Defense.

Dosage: Take 100 milligrams, three times a day with meals. (If you wish to take higher doses based on the research cited above, please discuss the matter with your doctor to avoid the risk of unwanted side effects.)

▮ GABA (Gamma-aminobutyric acid)

GABA is an amino acid that acts as a neurotransmitter in the central nervous system. It is essential for proper brain function. GABA is formed in the body from another amino acid, glutamic acid. Its function is to decrease neuron activity and inhibit nerve cells from overfiring.

At proper levels, it prevents anxiety and stress messages from reaching the brain by occupying their receptor sites. Too much GABA can cause increased anxiety, shortness of breath, numbness around the mouth, and tingling in the extremities.

Dosage: Take 500 milligrams daily, or follow package directions.

▮ Glutathione

Glutathione is often depleted in people with PD. It is a protein produced in the liver from the amino acids cysteine, glutamic acid, and glycine. It is a powerful antioxidant that neutralizes oxygen molecules before they can harm cells. Together with selenium, it forms the enzyme glutathione peroxidase, which neutralizes hydrogen peroxide. In addition to protecting individual cells, glutathione also defends the tissues of the arteries, brain, heart, immune cells, kidneys, lenses of the eyes, liver, lungs, and skin against oxidative damage.

Glutathione deficiency has been linked to nervous system problems, including lack of coordination, mental disorders, tremors, and difficulty with balance. Low levels of glutathione have been associated with Lewy body disease and may be an early indication of loss of brain cells in the substantia nigra. While the mechanism is not perfectly understood, researchers believe the low levels of glutathione do not directly cause cell death, but they make the cells more susceptible to toxic or free-radical exposure. Studies have found that treatment with glutathione has had benefits on Parkinson's symptoms.

Dosage: Supplemental glutathione can be expensive, so many experts recommend that you supply the body with the compounds it needs to make the nutrient. In other words, take glutathione, following package directions, or provide the body with the raw materials to make it on its own by taking 500 milligrams of N-acetyl cysteine daily.

▌ Vitamin B Complex

B vitamins are essential for healthy brain function and enzyme activity. In the body, the B vitamins are converted into agents necessary for proper brain and nervous system functioning though a process known as methylation. When a person experiences B vitamin deficiency, the process is inhibited and neurological problems develop.

Dosage: Take 50 milligrams of B complex twice a day with meals.

▌ Strive for a Toxin-Free Lifestyle ▌

Once your have been diagnosed with Parkinson's disease, it is essential that you minimize your exposure to pesticides, herbicides, and other chemical toxins. The substantia nigra in your brain has already experienced damage from a battle with environmental toxins, and you need to reduce the toxic load as much as possible.

- If you live or work in an environment where you have frequent exposure to toxins, consider moving or changing jobs, if possible.
- Drink purified, filtered water; do not drink well water.
- Choose organic foods whenever possible. Of course, organic foods are often more expensive than nonorganic foods, and for those of us on a fixed income, it can be a strain on the budget to spend extra. Try to slowly integrate some organic foods into your shopping list, starting with fruits and vegetables.

The supplements and eating strategies discussed in this chapter are considered beneficial for people with Parkinson's, but there is no standard supplement regimen. If you're interested in minimizing your symptoms using nutritional supplements, I recommend you work with a holistic physician, nutritionist, or herbalist to develop a customized plan.

▌ Eating Well

Generally, PD patients should eat a well-balanced diet, high in fruits and vegetables and relatively low in protein (problems with protein are discussed on p. 109). While there is no widely accepted Parkinson's diet with proven benefits, the following eating guidelines may help people with PD avoid or minimize some of their symptoms:

▌ *Eat more fiber.* Fiber prevents constipation (a common problem for people with Parkinson's) and it speeds food through the digestive tract, minimizing the time the food stays in the intestines. (Toxins that remain in the digestive tract can be absorbed into the bloodstream.) Most people eat about 15 grams of fiber daily; strive to consume at least 30 grams. To add fiber to your diet, eat whole fruits—especially prunes and dried fruits—and switch from refined to whole grains. If you still can't get enough fiber into your diet, consider a fiber supplement. When you switch to a high-fiber diet or supplement, add them to your diet slowly over time, in order to minimize temporary side effects, which could include gas, cramps, and diarrhea. I find that it helps me relax in the evening and aids in regularity for me to have a bowl of high-fiber cereal shortly before going to bed.

▋ *Drink plenty of water.* Water not only helps prevent constipation, it also helps with our respiratory systems, lubricates joints, and flushes waste from the bloodstream. Some Parkinson's medication can contribute to dehydration, so avoid complications by drinking at least eight 8-ounce glasses of filtered or bottled water daily.

▋ *Take probiotics.* These "good" bacteria found in yogurt with live cultures and supplements help complete the digestive process, reduce inflammation, and balance the endocrine system. Probiotic supplements often contain acidophilus bacteria; they are available at health food stores and some pharmacies.

▋ *Avoid spicy foods.* Some people with Parkinson's find that they experience violent dyskinesia after they eat spicy foods. If you recognize this pattern, skip the hot sauce and go bland.

▋ *Consume foods high in calcium, magnesium, and vitamin D.* People with Parkinson's are susceptible to thinning bones caused by osteoporosis. Orange juice with added calcium and dairy products (timed to avoid conflicting with medication, see pp. 109–110) can reduce your risk of brittle bones.

In addition, you will need to watch your calorie intake to reach and maintain a healthy weight. Some people with Parkinson's lose weight (tremors and dyskinesia can burn large numbers of calories);

others gain weight (some medications, especially those for depression, can cause weight gain). You may need to work with a nutritionist to develop a meal plan that provides an adequate diet based on healthy food choices.

▌ The Problem with Protein

After several years on levodopa-carbidopa, about half of all people with Parkinson's find that the drug begins to wear off before they are scheduled for another dose. When this happens, a person cycles between on and off periods as the level of medication in the bloodstream fluctuates.

This problem can become worse when a person eats protein-rich foods, such as meat or cheese. Take it from me, the South Beach and Atkins diets are not for us. In the digestive tract, protein is broken down into amino acids. Levodopa is also an amino acid, and it must compete with the other amino acids for a chance to be absorbed. When this happens, it may take longer for the levodopa to work, the drug may be less effective, or it may wear off more quickly. Furthermore, carbohydrates tend to speed absorption of levodopa into the brain.

Of course, you don't want to cut protein from your diet entirely—it's necessary for good health—but you do want to be strategic about eating it. Try to consume protein at least one hour before or after you take your medication (two hours is even better). Another tip is to eat carbohydrate-rich meals during the day and restrict protein to the evening meal when you're home for the day and may be less bothered by an increase in symptoms.

If you are like many of us and find that you must take your medication with some food in your stomach, try to make it something like crackers or a piece of bread. I do know one person who only felt right if he took his medication with milk. While milk contains proteins, he drank such a small amount—just enough to coat the way down for his medication—that it was not an issue for him.

Another approach is to balance your protein and carbohydrates at a ratio of about 7 grams of carbohydrate to 1 gram of protein. If you like to have small amounts of protein throughout the day, this eating plan may be preferable. With this approach you would consume more of your food in the form of healthy carbohydrates (fruits, vegetables, and whole grains), with a small amount of protein (meat, eggs, and dairy products). You may wish to consult a dietician with expertise in meal planning for more help.

Good nutrition and the wise use of supplements can provide your body with the nutritional support to combat Parkinson's. Frankly, there are no guarantees that the supplements and dietary changes listed in this chapter will dramatically reduce your symptoms and slow the progress of the disease, although there is theoretical evidence that they may. Eating a balanced diet and taking supplements to make up for any deficiencies in your diet will enhance your overall health, even if they don't offer a magic bullet for Parkinson's disease.

In addition to improved nutrition, you may benefit from other lifestyle changes as well. The following chapter discusses the importance of attitude and the benefits of mind-body techniques to change your mind-set about the disease.

9

Imagine:
The Importance of Attitude
and the Mind-Body Connection

Several years ago, Karen, 52, felt isolated, unable to talk to anyone who understood what she was going through with her Parkinson's disease. She didn't share the same concerns as the older people she met at her local support group, but ultimately she discovered the Movers & Shakers online discussions. "I finally found a group of people who really knew what I was going through," she said. "We had lots of late-night conversations, and I didn't feel so alone."

"I met Jim in the chat room. He was funny and so uplifting. He was always trying to get people to stop complaining and see the lighter side of PD," Karen R. said. "When Jim talked about his Parkinson's, he said, 'This is the way my book was written, it's up to me to deal with it.' I really envied that about him: he had a great attitude and made me feel I could be happy again, too. He told me, 'There will be ruts in the road, but you have to keep driving your car. That's the only way you'll get anywhere.' He always signed his e-mails 'Keep smiling.' His attitude was very attractive to me."

Over several months, their online relationship grew more personal. Karen and Jim met in 2003 and were married several months later. "We just meshed. When I hugged him, I fit right under his arm; we fit together perfectly," she said. "It was amazing. We're the best support we can be for each other. Sometimes we have pity parties, but then we think about how we can make ourselves stronger."

Like Karen and Jim, many people with Parkinson's can change the course of their lives by changing the way they look at the world. Attitude isn't everything, but it's a lot, especially when it comes to handling a chronic, debilitating illness.

As mentioned earlier, from the time of diagnosis, a person with Parkinson's must work through a wide range of emotions. No one should expect to be cheerful and positive about Parkinson's at first, of course, but so many aspects of life will go more smoothly if you are able to work through your feelings and make the best of your situation. I still have down days—trust me, more than I care to admit—but I do my best to let the negative feelings pass through me so that I can reclaim a positive perspective.

Having a positive outlook not only helps me see the good things that I still cherish in my life, but it also helps lower my stress level—and that has a direct impact on my Parkinson's disease. During times of stress and anxiety, my symptoms almost invariably flare. My tremors may become more pronounced; my speech may become weaker; my balance may be off. Sometimes when Michael is speaking to a group, he will get so excited that the adrenaline shoots through his body, his throat closes up and it's as if he's trying to force the air out to make his words heard. This can happen with "good stress"—such as a birthday party or going out for the night—as well as "bad stress"—such as when the car breaks down or the kids are sick or fighting.

In fact, studies have found that stress can indeed increase neuron loss in some brain regions of people with PD. Researchers at the University of Pittsburgh found that during times of stress, the body secretes hormones to weather the stressful episode, but that these same hormones at excessively high levels can become neurotoxic and promote cell death. Sounds scary, but the take-home message is clear: minimize stress as much as you can.

▪ How Stress Hurts

Over the past 30 years or so, scientists have studied the neurological links between the mind and the body. They have found that when faced with stress, the body's fight-or-flight response kicks in, unleashing a number of biochemical changes in preparation for dealing with danger.

When people with Parkinson's experience stress, our adrenaline surges and our bodies utilize dopamine differently. We metabolize dopamine faster and we often experience an intensification of our Parkinson's symptoms. "Stress is a killer," said Karen M., 56. "The moment stress begins, I start to tremor more, whether or not I've had medication. Stress is more powerful than any medication; it renders any medication ineffective."

I have the same response to stress. If I feel startled or surprised, I feel a shock shoot through my system and my tremors may go out of control. I need to do deep breathing before I can get myself settled, and in that short time I have literally spent a good portion of my available dopamine. That may mean that my latest dose of medication is less effective, and I may experience more symptoms.

Michael noticed a direct relationship between his stress level and Parkinson's symptoms when he was working in the insurance industry. He tried deep breathing and other ways to relax. Ultimately, he changed jobs to minimize his stress, although it's virtually impossible to avoid all stress when working any kind of job. (He now walks and goes fishing when he feels stressed.)

Fortunately, the stress response can be quickly reversed. Your body begins to relax as soon as your brain receives the signal that it's safe to calm down. About three minutes after the brain cancels the emergency signals to the central nervous system, relaxation begins.

People with Parkinson's must learn ways to manage stress, and we've got to give ourselves permission to opt out of some activities that can cause stress—even positive stress. I love the holidays, but it can be an exhausting and overwhelming time of year. When I decorate for Christmas, I can't deal with 12 boxes of decorations at once; the stress is too much. I need to slow down and do just one box at a time. We also need to be able to ask for help when we need it—and that isn't easy for some of us to do.

■ Mind-Body Stress Reduction Techniques

Life is stressful for everyone, particularly those of us with PD. Just as your body can't tell the difference between real and imagined stress, your body can't tell whether the relaxation response was triggered by a change in circumstances or a change in your attitude. This can work to your advantage because you can learn to promote relaxation and reverse the stress response by using various mind-body techniques.

Studies have shown that people who are well-trained in mind-body techniques can voluntarily lower their blood pressure and heart rate, alter their brain-wave activity, reduce blood-sugar levels, and ease muscle tension. With practice, you, too, can put mind over illness and use stress-reduction techniques to help control your Parkinson's symptoms.

This chapter will explore some of the many mind-body relaxation techniques. You can learn more about each approach by checking books out of the local library or contacting a community center or health clinic to inquire whether classes are offered in your area.

Biofeedback

Biofeedback involves training yourself to use your mind to voluntarily control your body's internal systems. You may be able to use the technique to relax your muscles, to get "unstuck" if you freeze, or to calm yourself in a crisis.

I have used this approach myself. I periodically experience times when I choke and feel my airway close down, even though there is nothing in my throat. I used to panic, unable to gasp for air, certain that I was going to die. After surviving several of these episodes, I learned that the best way to control these spasms is to remain calm. Even though every ounce of my being wants to scream and thrash about, I know that I need to relax and center myself until the moment passes and I can breathe normally. I have, in essence, learned to reprogram my response to these very frightening choking attacks.

My experience with self-calming did not involve formal training, but you can learn to short-circuit your stress by using biofeedback training. Almost anyone can learn the technique, but it takes practice. It's easy to get stressed out, but much more difficult to learn to relax. To learn the skill, you must be able to measure your physical state. Biofeedback machines are used by many holistic doctors and psychologists. There are personal units available for at-home use, but I would recommend working with a professional initially.

During a biofeedback session, electrodes are attached to various parts of your body to measure your heart rate, breathing, perspiration, pulse, blood pressure, temperature, muscle tension, and brain-wave patterns. The electrodes' wires are connected to a small machine that displays the data, usually in the form of pictures, graphic lines, or audible beeps. Using this information, you can literally watch yourself relax or grow tense, depending on certain stimuli.

Within bounds, you can actually learn to control your body's internal processes by carefully studying the measurable changes in your body as you relax and change your thought patterns. Once you learn to adjust your physical state to promote relaxation, you can do it without the biofeedback equipment.

Breathing

Deep breathing helps to relax the body and quiet the mind. Unfortunately, when we are stressed, most of us don't breathe fully. Instead of inhaling deeply and drawing in plenty of oxygen, we take shallow, rapid, weak breaths, filling only the top part of the lungs. This so-called chest breathing, or thoracic breathing, fails to adequately oxygenate the blood, making it more difficult to manage stress.

The preferred way of breathing is abdominal breathing, or diaphragmatic breathing. This type of breathing draws air deeply into the lungs, allowing the chest to fill with air and the belly to rise and fall. Newborn babies and sleeping adults naturally practice abdominal breathing, although most adults lapse into chest breathing during their waking hours. Having sung in a choir most of my life, this type of breathing comes very naturally to me, thanks to my many choir teachers who forced me to practice it again and again.

To relieve stress, become aware of your breathing and inhale more fully; you will immediately be able to feel the muscle tension and stress melt away in response to the improved oxygenation in your tissues. I find that a few deep breaths can help me feel calm and more ready to face a particular challenge, whether it's visiting a congressman's office on Capitol Hill to talk about Parkinson's legislation or trying to make it to the bathroom when my muscles are knotted when I wake up in the middle of the night. Concentrated deep breathing can help calm you and relieve stress at any time and in any situation. Of course, don't overdo it or you will hyperventilate. If you experience shortness of breath, heart palpitations, or a feeling that you can't get enough air when practicing deep breathing, stop immediately and return to your normal breathing pattern.

Creative Therapy

Creative therapies—including dance, music, and art—promote healing through the release of creative energy. One study reported in 1998 found that a group of PD patients who received 13 weekly two-hour music therapy sessions had better motor function than those who didn't have the musical outlet. The study showed that music therapy had a beneficial effect on the emotional functions, activities of daily living, and quality of life of Parkinson's patients.

It seems that the creative process—be it painting, drawing, singing, or playing the banjo—somehow relies on different pathways in the brain than those used for everyday activities, so that many people with Parkinson's find that their symptoms disappear when they are involved in their creative pursuit. The tremors disappear when the painter picks up a brush; the slowness vanishes when the dancer glides across the floor. In fact, many people with Parkinson's find that if they become stuck in a doorway or trying to turn a corner, they can sometimes get moving again by thinking of the movement as a dance step, rather than as walking from one side of the room to another.

In addition, some researchers have raised the possibility that PD and the medications used to treat it may contribute to the creative drive itself. Other researchers have reported newly developed artistic skills after starting treatment for PD, raising questions—but not yet answers—about the neurology of the artistic process.

Expressing Your Emotions

When diagnosed with PD or any other chronic medical problem, many people feel depressed, stressed, and angry—emotions that can make matters worse by further compromising the immune system. These feelings are to be expected, though you should try to take steps to work through them so that they do not further undermine your health. Experience has taught me that I can often decide to be happy or decide not to let my Parkinson's get me down; on those upbeat days, I almost always experience more joy and more humor than on the days when I let the dark cloud follow me through the day. Don't underestimate the power of learning to laugh at yourself.

Openly discussing the emotional side of illness can help many people resolve their negative feelings. Some people find it helpful to talk things over with a friend or loved one, while others appreciate the assistance of a professional counselor or a support group for people who share a similar medical problem. For information on support groups, see Chapter 12.

Laughter

Laughter produces endorphins, the feel-good hormones, which go a long way toward improving mood and general outlook on life. There is a close relationship between dopamine and endorphins; the more we laugh, the more we produce endorphins, which allow the dopamine we have to work more effectively. It's okay to laugh, even if you have Parkinson's; you need to enjoy yourself and have a good time despite this illness.

Find ways to bring joy into your life, whether it's spending time with your grandchildren, watching funny movies, or just joking around. The more we laugh, the better we feel.

Massage

Massage is a hands-on way of reducing stress that can be particularly helpful to people with PD because it can help to relieve some joint and muscle stiffness, reduce stress, and increase feelings of well-being. Some studies have shown that massage can naturally increase dopamine, the brain chemical that is depleted in Parkinson's disease.

Eight one-hour sessions of deep body massage over eight weeks resulted in improvement in self-confidence, well-being, walking and activities of daily living, according to a study done in the United Kingdom. A study at the University of Kansas found that weekly massage over a six-month period resulted in a 16 percent improvement in quality of life and a 29 percent improvement in depression, even though the participants actually experienced a progression of the Parkinson's symptoms. In other words, people's PD symptoms were worse, but they still reported feeling less depressed and more satisfied with their lives.

Massage stimulates the production of disease-fighting antibodies, and it reduces anxiety and stress-related hormones better than other muscle-relaxation techniques. Instead of making you feel drowsy, it can actually increase your alertness.

You can learn massage techniques yourself, either by checking out a book from the local library or by taking a class. You might also consider consulting a massage therapist, who should know a variety of techniques. Most states require licensing of massage therapists; if your state doesn't, look for a therapist with certification from a professional organization. For information on state licensing requirements and a list of certified massage therapists in your area, contact the National Certification Board for Therapeutic Massage and Bodywork at 800-296-0664 or www.ncbtmb.com.

Meditation

Though it comes in many different forms or traditions, meditation basically involves focusing your complete attention on one thing at a time. If you haven't tried it, meditation can feel strange at first. The mind tends to wander, and it can be a real challenge to maintain concentration when faced with a barrage of distracting thoughts. *Did I take my meds? Will I be able to make it to the graduation on Saturday?*

Meditation relieves stress because it is impossible to feel tense or angry when your mind is focused somewhere else. You can't experience negative thoughts—or the physiological responses to those thoughts—if your mind is tuned in to a neutral stimulus.

Studies have long supported the idea that meditation promotes relaxation. Research in 1968 at Harvard Medical School found that when people practiced transcendental meditation (TM; a type of mantra meditation), they showed physiological signs of deep relaxation. Their heart rate and breathing slowed, their oxygen consumption dropped by 20 percent, their blood lactate levels dropped, their skin resistance to electrical current increased, and their brain-wave patterns showed greater alpha-wave activity (the frequency associated with a state of deep relaxation).

More recent research has found that regular meditation can have notable effects on blood pressure, anxiety, chronic pain, body tension, and immune response and can clinically reduce cortisol levels, a measure of the body's stress level. Researchers have also shown, using magnetic resonance imaging (MRI), that meditation can activate certain structures in the brain that control the autonomic nervous system, a system that can become dysfunctional in some PD patients.

To experience the relaxing benefits of meditation, find a quiet place where you are not apt to be interrupted. Sit in a firm chair with your back as straight as possible, or lie down flat on your back on the ground. Then try one of the three basic types of meditation.

▌ *Mantra meditation* involves repeating—either aloud or silently—a word, a syllable, or a group of words each time you breathe out. I use prayer as my mantra. I find that when I take the time to be still and pray, it can ease many of my symptoms, even on the most horrid of days.

▌ *Gazing meditation* involves focusing both your attention and your gaze on an object such as a candle flame, a stone, or a flower. The object should be about one foot away from your face. Gaze at it rather than stare, keeping your eyes relaxed. Don't try to think about the object in words, just look at it without judgment.

▌ *Breathing meditation* involves focusing on the rise and fall of your breath. Draw a deep breath, focusing on the inhalation, the pause before you exhale, the exhalation, and the pause before you inhale. Each time you complete a breath and exhale, count 1 through 4, then start over with 1 when you exhale. The counting helps clear your mind of other thoughts.

No matter which type of meditation you choose, begin your session with a few minutes of deep breathing. When random thoughts enter your mind during your meditation time (as they almost certainly will), don't become anxious; just accept the thoughts and let them pass through your mind without notice or response. Start by meditating for 5 to 10 minutes once or twice a day, then work up to 15 to 20 minutes.

Progressive Relaxation

Progressive relaxation can produce a profound feeling of calm, as you systematically remove the stress from your body. Start by lying on your back on the floor, with your legs extended and your arms loose at your sides. Close your eyes and breathe deeply.

Once you are reasonably calm, begin to systematically tense and relax every muscle in your body. Start with your feet. Tense the muscles in your feet for 30 seconds or so, then relax them, allowing your feet to feel heavy and relaxed. Then move to your calves, thighs, abdomen, buttocks, hands, forearms, upper arms, shoulders, and face. When you finish, your muscles should feel soothed and relaxed. Lie quietly, and enjoy the feeling of complete relaxation.

Visualization

To relieve stress, use your imagination. Visualization—also known as guided imagery—builds on the idea that you are what you think you are. If you think anxious thoughts, your muscles will grow tense; if you think sad thoughts, your brain biochemistry will change and you will become unhappy. And more important, if you think soothing, positive thoughts, you will relax and develop a more positive outlook.

To experience the relaxation of visualization, sit in a comfortable position or lie on the floor in a quiet, dimly lit room. Tense all of your muscles at once, and hold for 30 seconds. Relax every muscle, and allow all the tension to drain from your body. Continue to inhale and exhale slowly and fully.

Once your muscles have relaxed, you can begin the visualization or imagery. First, concentrate on your breathing, feeling the regular rhythm of each breath and clearing your mind of all thoughts. Then imagine that you are in a peaceful setting, such as lying in the warm sun on a sandy beach or strolling down a country road on a cool October afternoon. Get all of your senses involved in your image. Smell the ocean mist, hear the leaves crunch under your feet. The more specific your fantasy, the more real it will seem. And the more real it seems, the more you will relax. Enjoy this "escape" for about 20 minutes. When you return to your body and get on with the challenges of the day, you will probably feel much more relaxed and refreshed.

■ Everyday Distractions from Stress ■

- Go fishing (that's Michael's favorite).
- Play video games (that's Gretchen's favorite).
- Play with the dog—or any other animal.
- Take a walk.
- Hunt for shells on the beach.

- Watch a movie, especially something funny.
- Wrestle or get physical.
- Put on some uplifting music and practice singing or dancing—or simply put on some relaxing tunes and let the music calm you.

You can use guided imagery to visualize changes in your physical state. You can visualize your muscles relaxing and your joints smoothly gliding through a full range of motion.

It's important to acknowledge that we aren't our disease. Too often we allow our diagnosis to define who we are and what we are capable of doing. These self-limiting thoughts can stop us in our tracks if we allow them to; instead, we must rise above those thoughts. We must be willing to laugh, to not feel obligated to live up to everyone else's expectations of us, while at the same time refusing to lower our own expectations of what we want to make of our lives.

While these and other relaxation techniques can be used to control your daytime stress levels, they can also be employed to get you in the right frame of mind for a restful night's sleep. It's difficult—if not impossible—to have a good rest if you're feeling anxious and stressed at bedtime. In the next chapter we look at the importance of rest and relaxation and the challenges people with Parkinson's face when trying to get enough sleep.

10

Replenish Yourself: The Importance of Rest and Relaxation

Parkinson's disease is exhausting. I haven't had a good night of sleep in the past seven years. I usually don't have too much trouble falling asleep, but I wake up after two or three hours and can't get back to sleep. I used to stare at the ceiling and feel frustrated and anxious, but I've learned to accept life as a night owl. I don't like alternating between sleepless nights and sleepy days, but I try not to beat myself up about it anymore.

Researchers report that at least half of all people with Parkinson's have trouble with sleep—although I'm surprised that the number isn't higher. Most people I know with PD suffer through the night. I can enter a Parkinson's chat room at any hour of the day or night and there is always someone online to talk to. For many of us, the Internet is a lifeline when the rest of the world seems to be asleep.

Now, I must acknowledge that being awake and being coherent are two different things. In the wee hours of the morning, I am often awake, but exhausted; I can't sleep, but I can't think straight, either. I've been known to talk nonsense—letting the conversation wander into a side thought about chili dogs or something totally off the point—or to wake up and find my head on the keyboard because I've actually fallen asleep staring at the computer screen.

I've learned the hard way that fatigue creates stress and makes Parkinson's symptoms worse. When I'm tired, I get grumpy and short-tempered; I'm not always charming to be around. In addition, I tend to have more tremors and symptoms, and I come down with colds and whatever else is going around.

When I'm up at night, I try to make up for it by napping in the afternoon. Sometimes I limit myself to a half-hour power nap, but when I've had a couple of tough nights in a row, I let myself surrender to sleep and I snooze as long as my body needs to. I am no longer a slave to the traditional nighttime sleep hours; my goal is to get the rest my body needs, whatever the time of day or night.

Even with an afternoon nap, I am often tired—and sometimes flat-out exhausted—during the day. It can be said that people with PD have two sleep-related problems: sleeping at night and staying awake during the day. In this chapter we look at both of these problems.

▌ Getting Enough Sleep at Night

The low dopamine levels caused by Parkinson's disease interfere with regular sleep patterns. People with PD often have trouble falling asleep, waking frequently during the night, and staying up for hours in the middle of the night. This condition is known as sleep fragmentation. Just as people with Parkinson's have good days and bad, we also have good nights and bad.

"Rest is a problem," said James, 51. "I suffer from insomnia. I get about two to three hours of sleep a night; sometimes I'm up for two or three days at a time. I've gotten used to it. If I get more than four hours of sleep, I feel stiff, almost frozen. It takes two doses of medication before I'm up and able to move enough to do anything.

About a month ago, I slept 12 hours, and it took almost 24 hours to get over that."

Sometimes we can blame the Parkinson's symptoms. It's hard to sleep through a muscle spasm or cramp. Some people with Parkinson's find that their bodies quiet down at night, saving the tremors for morning; others are awakened by the twitching and quivering of the bedsheets after the medication has worn off. Sometimes muscle aches and pains make it impossible to get comfortable, no matter how soft and supportive the mattress may be. Muscle rigidity can affect the bladder, leading to frequent trips to the bathroom throughout the night. Trust me, there's no rest for the weary.

Many people with PD suffer from a condition known as restless-leg syndrome. The name tells it all—when you're lying in bed at night, your legs feel restless and fidgety; you desperately want to get up and walk around. Some people also report feeling a creeping or crawling sensation in their legs. The restlessness goes away when you move, but it typically returns when you lie down again. I am sometimes able to outsmart my legs by taking a warm bath and then shuffling off to bed as soon as I get out of the water. (If I take a side trip to the bathroom or to the kitchen, my legs seem to wake up and feel restless again.)

People with Parkinson's sometimes suffer from REM Sleep Behavior Disorder (RSBD). These lively bedfellows physically act out their dreams, often kicking, screaming, sitting up, or walking around while asleep. As you might imagine, this condition can result in injury to the people with PD or anyone else around. Sometimes people with Parkinson's roam the neighborhood in their sleep, which can present its own set of hazards, especially for older people.

RSBD afflicts people with and without PD, but some researchers believe the two conditions could be linked. A study published in March 2006 in the journal *Neurology* found that RSBD could serve as an early marker of PD; studies estimate that approximately half of patients with RSBD will eventually develop PD. (The researchers observed this link, but did not explain how RSBD and PD may be related.)

Of course, medications can affect sleep, too. In an ironic twist, most drugs for PD bear warning labels indicating that they may cause drowsiness, yet they also tend to cause insomnia—you'll be sleepy and tired, but unable to fall asleep, which more or less sums up the nighttime hours for many of us. Sinemet and many anti-depressant medications can cause nightmares or vivid dreams that may interfere with a restful night's sleep.

In addition, as we get older, we awaken more often than we used to, and we spend more time fully awake in the middle of the night whether or not we have Parkinson's disease. Sleep studies have found that by age 65, most people wake up at least a dozen times a night and spend only about half an hour in the most restful periods of deep sleep. A 20-year-old, on the other hand, snoozes virtually without waking and accumulates about two hours of high-quality deep sleep.

Interestingly, people with Parkinson's who have had deep brain stimulation surgery tend to sleep better than those who have not had surgery. A study reported in the April 2006 issue of the *Journal of Neurology* found that DBS increased total sleep time and re-duced sleep problems for up to 24 months after treatment. Despite reduction in the use of medication, DBS did not reduce excessive daytime sleepiness.

Michael L., 48, sleeps better since he had DBS. "After the sur-gery, I started sleeping better than I had my entire life," he said. "I've dreamed dreams that were so real I didn't want to wake up. Sleep is enjoyable now. The nights used to be so long, and now they go by so fast."

Ultimately, it's up to you to determine if you have a sleep prob-lem. Our sleep demands change throughout our lives. If you're get-ting less sleep than you used to a few years ago, but you feel rested during the day, you don't have a problem. On the other hand, if you're tired during the day, you aren't getting enough rest, regardless of how many hours you spend in bed.

■ Tips to Get More Sleep

You may feel you've already tried everything possible to improve your sleep. Here are a few more ideas to try:

■ Try melatonin. A study published in September 2005 in the journal *Sleep Medicine* found people taking 50 milligrams of melatonin daily had more efficient sleep compared to those taking a placebo.

■ Limit your caffeine intake. You already know that too much caffeine, especially late in the day, can keep you awake at night. Opt for decaf in the evening.

■ Save your bed for sleeping and sex. Don't eat, watch TV, or read in bed. (Frankly, I have a TV in my bedroom and often snooze in front of the tube, but many sleep experts swear that you will fall asleep more easily if you train your mind to expect to sleep when you crawl under the covers.)

■ Make sure your bedroom is dark, quiet, and well ventilated. You want to minimize distractions and maximize comfort.

■ Don't be a slave to the clock. Go to bed when you feel tired, not when you think you should sleep.

■ Skip the nightcap. A single glass of wine or beer may help you relax at the end of the day, but don't overdo it. Having a couple of drinks before turning in may make you feel tired, but the alcohol may interfere with getting a good night's sleep. In addition, alcohol may interact with medication and intensify the drowsiness that is a side effect of some medications.

■ Exercise regularly. Working out helps improve sleep; just don't exercise in the several hours before bed.

▌ Don't go to bed with a full stomach. Overeating before bed can trigger heartburn or indigestion, as well as insomnia. If you need a snack, keep it light.

▌ If you're feeling hungry before bed, have a small snack. Try some warm chamomile tea.

▌ Take a short nap. Taking a half-hour cat nap can make you feel refreshed without reversing your day and night sleep cycles. I confess: if I'm worn out and haven't slept for days, I will snooze as long as I can. There are times I just can't push myself through the fatigue, and I give in to it. I will, however, opt for the brief nap instead of the marathon sleep session if I'm not exhausted.

▌ Talk to your doctor. In some cases you may find that prescription medications can help you get a good night's sleep. (In my limited experience, sleeping pills can help you get to sleep, but they don't help you stay asleep for the entire night.)

▌ Staying Awake During the Day

The inevitable consequence of not sleeping at night is being tired during the day. I don't do it often, but I have been known to nod off during the day in the middle of a conversation. For some of us, the problem occurs often enough to earn the label "day-night reversal" because our sleep patterns have been inverted. This can be particularly difficult for people who are working full-time and need to live by the demands of the alarm clock. It's tough to wake up ready for the day when you spent the night tossing and turning, only to doze off two hours before the alarm sounds.

Driving long distances can present a serious danger to some people with Parkinson's, especially those prone to "sleep attacks"—narcolepsy, or unexpected periods of sudden sleep. I've fallen asleep in the checkout line at Sam's Club and while singing at choir rehearsal.

Many people who are vulnerable to sleep attacks find it difficult to stay awake while driving. We recommend that you not drive long distances alone; have someone else in car with you to share the driving and to keep you company. Never drive if you are feeling drowsy or spacey; you're probably not going to be a good judge of just how tired you really are.

Talk to your doctor if daytime sleepiness proves to be a problem. You may be able to feel more alert by adjusting the dosage or timing of your medication. In some cases, your doctor may want to prescribe a medication to make you feel more awake. I don't recommend getting into a habit of taking one pill to get to sleep and another to stay awake, but you should discuss the matter openly with your doctor.

Your doctor may want to refer you to a clinic for a sleep study. I've had two sleep studies. In the first one, I had no REM sleep; I never made it to the deeper, more restful stages of sleep. In the second one, I had about 20 minutes of deep REM sleep. This isn't enough. If you can't sleep, you can't dream. Without dreaming you can't let go of all of the things you need to let go of in your dreams.

You may be able to enhance your nighttime sleep by working on relaxation during the day. Consider tai chi, yoga, meditation, massage, and other forms of relaxation. Increased stress can increase the intensity of tremors and other Parkinson's symptoms.

Poor sleep on an ongoing basis can change your outlook on life, leaving you depressed as well as exhausted. You may lose interest in doing things that once brought you joy, feeling that you lack both the physical and emotional strength to be the person you once were. You need to take whatever steps you can to rest and rejuvenate your body on a daily basis, but you also need to be willing to seek help for depression if the need arises. Working through depression is discussed in Chapter 11.

11

Experience Joy: The Importance of Treating Depression

This dreaded disease! It takes and takes and keeps on taking. I spent another night in pain. I shake and tremble in the dark of night, pillows and blankets tossed on the floor. Meds seem useless as the ringing alarm sounds time for another round. It's 2:00 A.M.—or is it 3:00? It really makes no difference. Powerless to escape its stranglehold on my body, I cry and whimper in the darkness. I cry out to my God and begin to wonder if he hears me. These are some of the worst days I've seen.

I am slipping away, replaced by an empty shell of a man. What once was is almost gone. At 43, my life seems so meaningless. I don't like saying these things, nor do I welcome these thoughts. I keep fighting but I feel victory slipping away. I feel powerless to stop time or at least slow its effect on my body. My greatest desire is simply to be able to sleep and to stop hurting.

Michael posted these words at 5 A.M. one morning on the Movers & Shakers online discussion group. Like so many of us, he needed to express his despair so that he could allow it to pass through him. The darkness can take over if you're not willing to acknowledge and confront it. Michael's e-mail continued:

> *I am far from giving up, just tired of hurting and needing to sleep. Tomorrow is another day, and I will make the best of it with what strength, talent, personality, skills, abilities, knowledge, and wisdom I have left so that those that follow will know there is hope, encouragement, and love among you.*

Michael is not alone in his sadness. Experts report that major depression is present in about 40 percent of Parkinson's patients at any given time, with a lifetime incidence of as much as 90 percent. While that figure may seem astoundingly high, it doesn't really surprise me. In my experience of working with people with Parkinson's disease, I believe that most of us do experience depression at some point, although some are loathe to admit it. In my opinion, the stigma against depression is alive and well within the Parkinson's community, especially among men. I wish it were different, but I know quite a few men—and a few women—who stubbornly refuse to acknowledge their depression. Perhaps they feel their bodies have already betrayed them and they cannot accept that their minds may do so as well. In any case, I wish that everyone with depression could feel comfortable seeking the help they need. Parkinson's disease diminishes the dopamine supply, which affects mood as well as movement. Depression is not a sign of weakness, and seeking help for depression is a sign of strength and good health.

▌ Parkinson's and Depression

Though many people confuse the two, depression isn't the same as sadness. While we all feel sadness in response to certain situations—the death of a loved one, the loss of a job, a divorce, or some other disappointment—depression is characterized by ongoing feelings of worthlessness, pessimism, sadness, and lack of interest in life. With clinical depression those feelings linger for weeks or months and ultimately become incapacitating.

Depression can be either a minor short-term problem or a lifelong, life-threatening illness. In fact, more than four out of five people who commit suicide are depressed, and the suicide rate among older people is three to four times higher than the rate for the general population.

Parkinson's can sometimes be confused with depression, especially early in the course of the disease. For example, the loss of facial expression may be mistaken for a depressed appearance, and the slowness and stooped posture of people with PD may be mistaken for the weary appearance of someone who is depressed.

▌ Factors Contributing to Depression

People with Parkinson's face several different, overlapping factors that contribute to depression.

▌ *Situational depression.* Living with Parkinson's means living with a body that doesn't work the way it once did. You're facing a lifetime with a chronic, degenerative neurological disease that has no cure; in other words, you've got a reason to feel frustrated and demoralized. This disease is life-altering, and anyone diagnosed with it will experience some change in his or her outlook, whether the disease is progressing slowly or rapidly.

▌ *Biochemical depression.* The same disease that is robbing your brain of the dopamine required for smooth motor movement is also robbing your brain of the feel-good neurotransmitters required for a positive outlook on life; in other words, your brain chemistry is being altered, causing biochemical depression. Many people with PD experience depression before the other signs of PD take hold, perhaps reflecting a change in brain chemistry that shows up as depression even before the first tremor has a chance to rear its ugly head.

▌ *Motivational depression.* Many people with Parkinson's develop a general malaise or apathy that is similar to—but distinct from—depression. What once made you happy no longer holds your interest; rather than participate in your own life, you want to sit at home, draw the curtains, and shut out the world. Psychologists consider this apathy separate from depression; many of the medications used to treat depression do not relieve the apathy. (The antidepressant Lexapro and the over-the-counter nutritional supplement SAM-e do tend to help relieve the apathy.)

In addition, researchers have found that the severity of depression correlates to poor sleep quality and nightmares. In a study of 120 people with Parkinson's, researchers at Brown University found that more than half the study participants had nightmares and a third had other sleep disorders. Other studies have found that more than two-thirds of people with Parkinson's have some form of sleep disorder at some time.

While sleep problems, brain chemistry, apathy, and the day-to-day realities of Parkinson's can all come into play in triggering depression, I have noticed that most people with Parkinson's do experience depression to some degree. In my experience, most people hit what we lovingly refer to as "the wall" about two to three years after their initial diagnosis. That's about the point when you realize that the constant cycle of taking medications will never end. That's the point when many vulnerable marriages begin to crumble, when some people lose their jobs, when the irritating symptoms become more debilitating. The permanence of the situation becomes painfully evident: there is no relief; there is no escape.

The desire to help others get over the wall was one of the motivating factors for starting Movers & Shakers. Michael and I realized that the earlier people can get support and the more knowledge they receive about the illness, the less likely the wall will feel insurmountable.

Some people struggle more than others, but most of us end up feeling down now and then. This is a natural part of dealing with this disease. The key to overcoming the limitations of Parkinson's disease is to have the mind-set that you *will* overcome it. In addition, you must acknowledge that you may have some days when you feel overwhelmed and defeated—but that tomorrow is another day. Finally, you must accept help, whether in the form of medication, a support group, or a talk with a friend, and then keep on going. Depression and apathy can be treated. Please, please allow yourself to ask for and accept help.

Marian, 60, struggled with depression after her diagnosis with PD.

After I was diagnosed with Parkinson's, my doctor put me on several medications. For a long time, I didn't even know that one of the drugs was an antidepressant. When I found out what it was, I decided I didn't need it since I had never been depressed. Then I found out what depression really was.

I had no idea how dark things could be. I went to a dark place and I couldn't come out. It was not that oh-the-cake-fell-and-I-feel-bad kind of sadness; it was a there-can-never-be-a-party-with-a-cake-and-I'll-never-get-over-it kind of sadness. Overwhelming and hopeless.

Suicidal thoughts were part of it, too. If someone with Parkinson's tells me they don't have suicidal thoughts, I tell them they're lying. I take 12 pills every morning, and there have been plenty of days that I think about how easy it would be to swallow all of them at once. At least one out of every three of my friends with Parkinson's have had suicide attempts. We try to support each other and talk things through before it gets too bad.

There are still times when I'm stuck in bed for three days and I think, "What's the point in going on?" I try to remind myself that it's the lack of dopamine that's bringing me down. And then when I do get out and I encounter other people who are crabby and sarcastic, I tell myself, "They just need a little more dopamine."

▌Overcoming Apathy

Recently researchers have recognized that people with Parkinson's can be apathetic without being depressed; apathy may be a core characteristic of Parkinson's disease separate from depression. It can be difficult to differentiate between the two. Loss of motivation, loss of interest, loss of effortful behavior, neutral mood, and a sense of indifference dominate the list of characteristics of apathy.

Apathy can be an extremely debilitating symptom on its own, even if a person does not meet the traditional criteria for depression. Often apathy interferes with a person's ability to take steps to improve his or her life or manage the Parkinson's symptoms. A person who feels apathetic is not being lazy or difficult; the apathy may be a symptom of the Parkinson's disease.

According to the July 2006 issue of the journal *Neurology*, the current criteria for diagnosing depression may not be appropriate for people with Parkinson's. Instead, a doctor may need to screen separately for both apathy and depression.

Spouses are typically the first to recognize apathy, and this lack of enthusiasm can be very destructive to any relationship. "Why don't you have any energy for me?" is a common complaint among spouses of people with Parkinson's. However well-intentioned a family member may be, such comments only increase the feelings of guilt and blame that the person with Parkinson's may be feeling about inconveniencing other family members in the first place. This is a difficult disease and many families could benefit from group and individual counseling so that each person can understand the way the disease is affecting other family members.

Unfortunately, many doctors don't pick up on apathy as a condition that needs to be dealt with separately. Some medications that work to treat depression do not have any impact on motivational disorders. Research is underway to assess the impact of various medications on apathy, but in the meantime, be sure to discuss this issue with your doctor so that he or she can help you rediscover the joy of everyday living.

▌ Warning Signs

It can be difficult to tell the difference between clinical depression and common sadness. But there are certain warning signs.

- Changes in sleep—either insomnia or sleepiness
- Changes in weight and eating habits—either weight gain or weight loss
- Loss of sexual desire or libido
- Chronic fatigue or tiredness
- Low self-esteem or self-worth
- Loss of productivity at work, home, or school
- Inability to concentrate or think clearly
- Withdrawal or isolation
- Loss of interest in activities that were once enjoyable
- Anger, irritability, or bad mood
- Trouble accepting praise or affirmation
- Feeling slow; every activity takes supreme effort
- Apprehension about the future

■ Frequent weeping or sobbing
■ Thoughts of suicide or death

These are all warning signs and diagnostic criteria for depression. In addition, a person who is depressed may show decreased facial expression and walk with a stooped posture—symptoms similar to those associated with Parkinson's disease. If you or a loved one experience three or more of these symptoms for two weeks or longer, contact a doctor or mental health professional for help. Don't try to treat serious depression by yourself. And if you or someone you're concerned about feels suicidal, immediately seek help from a specialist or a twenty-four-hour hotline; look in the phone book under "Suicide Prevention."

Lila, 49, has occasionally considered suicide. "I thought about killing myself on several occasions," she said. "Once I decided to give up and stop taking my medication. I couldn't move from the couch for nine days. I decided that was a slow death, and I didn't want that either. I tell myself that this disease isn't going to get the best of me. If I'm not dying, I'd better get busy living."

■ Treatment for Depression

For most people with PD, depression is an organic illness involving physical and biochemical changes in the body; without help, these people cannot "snap out of it," no matter how hard they try. While counseling and professional care can be crucial in recovery, medication may be necessary, too.

When it comes to dealing with depression, most mental health professionals rely on three types of treatment—counseling (psychotherapy or talk therapy), medication (drug therapy), and electroconvulsive therapy (ECT or shock therapy). These techniques can be used alone or in combination. Because depression can be caused by a wide variety of factors working together, a combination approach is often most successful.

In most cases, depression responds relatively quickly to medications, such as drugs that inhibit the reuptake of serotonin (SSRIs), allowing the serotonin in the body to work longer. (The major drawbacks to SSRIs are possible weight gain and sexual dysfunction.) If you do try medication, give the drugs a chance to work. Antidepressants often take several weeks to lift symptoms of depression. Medication should be used for a month or two during an initial trial; if it doesn't work or if there are unwanted side effects, another antidepressant should be tried. The vast majority of people will find at least some relief from their depression if they work with their doctors to explore a range of treatments. Don't despair; try something else.

Note: Two medications used to treat depression and other mood disorders that should be avoided by people with Parkinson's disease are amoxapine and lithium; both of these drugs can exacerbate Parkinson's symptoms.

▌ Working Toward Acceptance

I try to warn people when they are first diagnosed that people with Parkinson's must repeatedly go through the stages of grieving identified by psychologist Dr. Elisabeth Kübler-Ross. It is essential that you allow yourself to ride the emotional roller coaster, to feel all of the emotions that surround your disease and its progression. Parkinson's disease may not be terminal, but you must go through the grieving process when you are first diagnosed, as well as during times you experience a setback in your condition.

The five stages of grief are identified as:

Stage 1:   Denial and isolation

Stage 2:   Anger
Stage 3:   Bargaining
Stage 4:   Depression
Stage 5:   Acceptance

Keep in mind that you can't reach the stage of acceptance until you've worked through the other stages. The challenge with Parkinson's disease—or any other degenerative disease—is that once you reach the stage of acceptance, you experience another setback or new symptoms that require that you start the process over again. You have to mourn the reality of the disease; you have to mourn the progression of your tremors; you have to mourn the loss of your job; you have to mourn the loss of your ability to walk without a cane or walker. People with PD must constantly adjust their worldview; we must be in a perpetual state of healing because there is no other choice.

This constant revolving door of grief is natural, but many people need help to keep moving and not get bogged down in depression. That's not always easy, I understand. Please don't be afraid to talk openly about your feelings with members of a support group and with your doctor. Many people with Parkinson's find benefit from antidepressant medications.

Too often men with PD try to be stoic and strong by denying their depression, but they would be better served by recognizing the real strength in facing their emotions and doing whatever is necessary to reclaim their lives, even if that means taking medication for depression. Without treating the depression, all you're doing is adding to your pain.

While you should work with your primary-care physician or neurologist to address any problems you may have with depression, you may find that support groups for people with Parkinson's can be very helpful in affirming your feelings and boosting your emotions. The following chapter provides background on working with a support group, as well as starting one on your own.

Michael's View from the Mountaintop

I went though a period of depression about five years ago. I was recently divorced, unemployed, almost broke, and I had just moved 300 miles away from home to make a fresh start. All of those realities followed me and then hit me like a ton of bricks. All I could do was crawl out of the rubble, get on my knees, and admit to God that I wasn't in control of my life anymore.

When a man loses everything—including his pride, self-esteem, and ego—then he discovers his true character. That is when I decided to get up and begin again. I accepted that I had PD. I realized that in my pursuit of material riches, I had missed out on life itself—the warm sun on my face, a cool breeze through my hair, raindrops on my tongue.

As I began my new life, one in which I accepted my Parkinson's, I discovered a new way of living. It was a celebration of life itself. I now invest in sunsets and bird songs, the feel of morning dew on my toes as I walk through the grass. Sometimes I am so overwhelmed by it all that I cry tears of joy; it took PD to awaken me to this world and all the glorious things God has given us. He has lifted me out of my valley of despair and placed me on the mountaintop. Friends, there is plenty of room up here, and the view is spectacular.

12

Talk: The Importance of Support Groups

For five years, Karen M., 56, kept her Parkinson's disease a secret. She struggled through her long days as a home health-care worker, then did her best to fill out the extensive paperwork using her tiny, almost illegible script.

"I was worse than some of the patients I helped take care of, but I felt ashamed and frightened," she said. "I was in the Parkinson's closet. I took my medication, but I didn't want to tell anyone; I wanted to deny it as long as I could."

Karen's condition grew worse, but she felt the need to carry the burden alone and in silence. Eventually she found the courage to join an Internet chat room. "I came alive again when I read about other people talking about the illness. It was the first time that I saw I didn't have to die with Parkinson's disease—I could continue to live.

"The people online were so open and honest. It became much easier to open up in the chat room. Everyone had Parkinson's. It was much harder to open up in my life with my friends and family, but I was able to take what I learned in the support group and bring some of that honesty into the rest of my life."

Many people with Parkinson's have found healing through the support of others. "Once I got with other people and I heard their stories of courage and faith, I found these encounters more beneficial than a visit to my neurologist," said Tom, 67. "My neurologist is looking at the disease as a doctor; the people I spoke with are living it every day."

Tom was able to draw strength from his encounters with other people who shared his diagnosis. "I didn't want to be a sick person. I didn't want to have a tremor or use a cane. I didn't want to look in the mirror and see an old person. In the group, I saw people with my same appearance but a different attitude. I saw positive people and I found the courage to change my attitude. They gave me new hope."

It doesn't matter how strong or well-balanced you are emotionally, you can benefit from some kind of PD support group. Being part of a group helps you connect with other people, it allows you to be heard and validated by people who really do understand what you are going through. By sharing your wisdom and experience with other people, you will become stronger. I can't tell you how many times I've been feeling blue and I've been called by someone else who feels even worse. Instead of focusing on my despair, I put my energy into lifting the other person up, and in turn, we both feel better by the end of the conversation. The gift I attempt to give the other person becomes a gift I also give to myself.

In addition, I've learned a lot about PD from other people in support groups. I've never been seen by a doctor who has PD, but I've spoken with hundreds of people who live with this disease on a daily basis. While my doctors can talk about the theoretical realities of managing Parkinson's, I've learned lots of practical information from the people who are living with the disease. What I learn I try to pass on—and that is one of the reasons I wanted to write this book.

If you're interested in a more pragmatic reason to join a support group, here it is: Studies have found that even people with fatal illnesses live far longer when they are part of a support group than those who did not participate in a support group.

▌ Finding a Support Group

There are a number of different types of support groups. Some are only for people with Parkinson's disease; others welcome anyone with a degenerative neurological disease (such as multiple sclerosis or Lou Gehrig's disease). Some Parkinson's groups focus on the concerns of people with the young-onset form of the disease; others encourage participation from people of all ages. Some groups focus on emotions and moral support; others bring in guest speakers and have an educational component. Some meet once a month; others gather once a week. There is no single "right" type of group; try a few and find out what type of experience feels best to you.

In addition, some groups meet face-to-face at a regular time and place, while others meet in cyberspace. Mover & Shakers as well as other national Parkinson's groups offer online discussion groups that include people from all over the country. Some people find it easier to open up on the computer, since they don't need to feel self-conscious about their tremors and dyskinesia. Online groups also allow the group to include a much broader number of participants; if you've got a computer with Internet service, you can connect with someone with Parkinson's 24/7. That can be a huge benefit if you find yourself pacing the floor at 3 A.M., unable to sleep and desperate to speak to someone about what you're feeling.

"I have contacted people in my support group in the middle of the night," said Lila, 49. "On a bad day, I sometimes need to talk to someone, just to say, 'I hate this; I can't do it anymore.' All it takes to help me is another voice saying, 'I understand' and I know that they do."

Studies have supported the finding that people benefit from participating in Parkinson's support groups. Researchers at the University of California looked at the effectiveness of online support groups for Parkinson's disease. A 20-week study involving 66 people with Parkinson's found that people who preferred online support groups were younger and less depressed, and had a higher quality of life, than PD patients in traditional support groups. Overall, the support-group participants showed improved quality of life, although they did not experience lower rates of depression.

The Internet can be an invaluable resource in finding support groups. Many hospitals and neurology clinics have support groups; ask your doctors about any groups that might meet in your area. The American Parkinson Disease Association, the National Parkinson Foundation, and the Parkinson's Disease Foundation all offer support groups nationwide. (For contact information for these groups, see the section on "Resources" at the end of the book.)

Many other people benefit from online support groups. "When I was first diagnosed, I isolated myself," said James, 51. "I was ashamed of my trembling and stumbling. For about a year, I did nothing. I didn't talk to my friends. I didn't interact with the world. I was depressed and learned about Parkinson's from the Internet. I started reading message boards, and I came away feeling I wasn't alone anymore."

Karen R. believes her life changed because of her participation in a Parkinson's support group. "Before I knew I had Parkinson's disease, I didn't know what I was here for," she said. "Had I not found the Parkinson's chat room, I would be in a different place in life. I think I've done a lot of good helping other people in the chat rooms. It has given me a purpose. I don't need as much support as I used to, but I still need to support other people."

▌ The Faces of Parkinson's

Attending your first support group meeting may be very difficult. For one thing, you may feel vulnerable and uncomfortable opening up emotionally in front of a group of strangers. In addition, you may look around you and see other people in far more advanced stages of the disease and find yourself wondering, "Is this my future?"

When a 42-year-old Alabama woman with YOPD went to her first support group meeting, she felt alone. "I looked around and all the people there were old. I cried; I felt like there was nobody like me in the world." She eventually learned to see beyond the gray hair and wrinkles and appreciate the similarities between her struggles and those of the older people in her support group, but her initial impression was distressing.

If you are in the process of accepting your initial diagnosis, you may have a great deal of fear and anxiety about what it means to live with Parkinson's disease. Before attending the group for the first time, you might ask about the age range of the participants, as well as how far the disease has advanced in most of the participants. If you are 42 and newly diagnosed, you may find it shocking and discouraging to sit down with people in their seventies and eighties in advanced stages of the disease; their physical condition may confirm all of your greatest fears about the disease. It must be noted, however, that even if someone at a meeting is shaking or twitching, he or she probably has a lot of interesting and important information to share if you're able to stay and listen.

I recommend that you have some sense in advance of who might attend the meeting so that you can mentally prepare yourself for the experience. There is a great deal you can learn from anyone in the group, but you can only hear what they have to say if you open yourself up to the experience. Alternatively, you may seek out groups designed for people newly diagnosed with Parkinson's or those who have young-onset Parkinson's. Again, there is no single arrangement that works for everyone, but to get the most out of the group, you might want to have some idea of what you will encounter before you attend.

▌ Special Needs for YOPD

While the diagnosis of Parkinson's disease can be devastating at any age, it presents unique challenges—both emotional and practical—to someone under age 50. The feelings of shock and denial can be difficult to dismiss; it seems the whole world is telling them, "You're too young to have Parkinson's."

It forces a person to rewrite a lifetime of plans. Younger people may have small children at home, 25 years left on a home mortgage, a career just starting to fall into place. What will happen to their marriage? How will they pay for the children's college? How long will they be able to work? In other words, there could be no less convenient a time to develop a degenerative neurological disease with no cure.

It can take some time for a younger person to realize that PD is not a death sentence, but it may demand some new visions of what the future will hold.

▌ Start Your Own Group

If you live in a community that does not currently have a Parkinson's support group or offers a group that does not meet your particular needs, consider starting one of your own.

For reasons of confidentiality, your doctor cannot give you the names of other Parkinson's patients. However, if you wish to share your name with other patients, your doctor can pass your contact information on to them.

The groups mentioned above have manuals and information for people interested in starting new support groups. Keep in mind that a spouse, a friend, or a family member can start a Parkinson's support group without having the disease. Free meeting space is often available at senior citizen centers, churches, synagogues, hospitals, and YMCA/YWCA organizations. Smaller groups might consider meeting at someone's home.

When I was first diagnosed and living in a rural town, I did not know anyone who lived near me who had Parkinson's disease, and I had never heard of anyone under age 50 who had it. I began to use the Internet to make connections, but I often found the chat rooms empty and posting notices on message boards didn't provide a chance for dialogue.

After several postings, I received an e-mail from a man with young-onset Parkinson's disease who lived in Florida. He wanted to start an online support group on AOL. I never imagined the changes that would happen in my life when I agreed to start a chat room with Michael.

We found that most Parkinson's disease websites focused on medical research and scientific studies. We both appreciated the need for research—we want a cure to be found for this disease—but we also wanted to talk about the here and now. Many people with Parkinson's need help today, and they need to connect with others who understand what they are going through in a personal way. We encountered people with Parkinson's who needed friendship—perhaps a discussion about something other than PD, a joke, or even a friendly voice over the telephone. Movers & Shakers was founded to fulfill some of those needs, as well as to provide information and support to those battling Parkinson's.

Members of Movers & Shakers provide emotional support for one another; we form, in essence, a community of mutual caregivers. We also recognize the importance of the caregivers who support us in our homes on a day-to-day basis, putting their love for us into action by helping us through the day in ways both large and small. Chapter 13 examines the importance of caregivers and it describes ways that we can support those who take care of us.

13

Taking a Break: The Importance of Caring for Your Caregivers

James, 51, learned he had Parkinson's disease six years ago, but he still struggles when he needs to ask for help; he is an unwilling care receiver because he wants to be able to take care of his family instead of the other way around.

> I want to be the breadwinner and the king of the castle, but I am the one being cared for and my wife is the caregiver. She works in the medical field and knows what's going on with me. She's good to me, but I have a problem with it. I don't like being disabled. I don't feel disabled—until the Parkinson's lets me know it's real.
>
> One of the hardest parts is disappointing my children. Sometimes I have a Parkinson's Day and I can't attend a school play or a basketball game. I'm not as reliable as I used to be. I see disappointment in my daughter's eyes; she's a worrywart, and she worries about her dad a lot.

Like James, many people with Parkinson's disease—including Michael and I—find it difficult to accept the limitations imposed by the disease; we find it more comfortable to give care than to receive it. We have a hard time asking for help. Part of this is due to the need to maintain some level of control over a life than sometimes appears to be out of control.

Michael and I have a unique perspective because we are both patients and caregivers to each other. At times I am the one who requires a little extra assistance; at other times, Michael needs a hand. Ultimately, however, virtually every person with Parkinson's disease will need support with daily activities. Good communication between the caregiver and care receiver can make the relationship between them much smoother.

Too often caregivers aren't given the respect and appreciation they deserve for taking on this significant responsibility. In most cases, the person with Parkinson's gets all the attention: How are you feeling? Did you rest last night? Do you need help with anything? The relationship between the caregiver and care receiver is often unbalanced and one-directional, which doesn't serve the needs of either party.

Being a caregiver isn't easy; it can be a stressful and daunting task, but it can also be very rewarding. This chapter will describe the challenges of caregiving and ways to care for your caregiver. Those of us with Parkinson's depend on those who help us, and we can't afford to lose them to sickness or burnout. We need to have two-way communication and time apart so that they can renew themselves and maintain a healthy perspective about the relationship.

▌ Tips for Caregivers

While by no means a comprehensive list, the following tips may help you avoid certain common pitfalls encountered by many caregivers.

▌ Don't surrender your life to your loved one with Parkinson's. You should not allow Parkinson's disease to take control of your life.

▌ Be good to yourself. Take time to read, go for a walk, practice a hobby, visit your friends. You are doing important—but difficult—work and you need some time for yourself.

▌ Sleep well.

▌ Exercise regularly. You need to exercise as much as we do.

▌ Be on the lookout for signs of depression. Don't be embarrassed to seek professional help if you think it would be beneficial.

▌ Let other people help you. When friends or family ask how they can be useful, make a specific suggestion of what they can do.

▌ Learn as much as you can about Parkinson's disease. The more you know what to expect and why we do what we do, the more you can understand the situation.

▌ Some tasks require physical strength and stamina. It can be difficult to help us in and out of cars, to push us in wheelchairs, or to lift us when we fall. Be willing to know when you can't perform a task without assistance.

▌ Don't do too much. It's important for people with Parkinson's to maintain our independence. Let us try to take care of ourselves as much as we can, but be there to back us up if we need help. It may take me 20 minutes to button my blouse, but it's important that I continue to control the things I can.

▌ Remember that your care receiver's needs may change from day to day or hour to hour. If we can move around easily one minute and not another, we are not being lazy; we may need a dose of medication or a period of rest. This is not personal.

▌ Be as patient as you can. People with Parkinson's move slowly and can take a frustrating amount of time to perform simple tasks. Remember, we're doing the best we can.

▌ Be ready for emergencies. Most caregivers have little or no training and may be unprepared to handle every emergency. Make a list of emergency contacts and post it by the phone so that you can ask for help if you need it.

▌ Allow yourself to grieve the loss of some dreams you may have had with your partner—then allow yourself to imagine new dreams.

▌ Accept your feelings. Having negative feelings—such as frustration or anger—about your responsibilities or the person for whom you are caring is normal. It does not mean you are a bad person or a bad caregiver. It does not mean that you do not love the person you are helping.

▌ Share your feelings and frustrations with other caregivers. You will benefit from knowing that you are not alone.

▌ Tips for Care Receivers

Care receivers must share the burden of establishing and preserving a good relationship with their caregivers. The following suggestions may help.

▌ We must learn to accept our disabilities. No one wants to remind us of our limitations, especially when we already know what they are but don't want to admit them.

▌ We should stop apologizing for our condition. Our caregivers know that we are not responsible for our disease; they just want to help us get through the day.

▌ We must remember to say "Thank you." A little gratitude can go a long way.

▌ Sometimes we need to put forth the extra effort to go out, even when we don't want to. Our caregivers need to get out of the house, and they appreciate when we try to join them.

- We need to do exercises on our own; it shouldn't be up to our caregivers to nag us about our routine.
- We should make every effort to communicate our feelings, without making our caregivers ask a lot of questions or act like detectives to figure out what is bothering us.
- We should remember that our caregivers are busy with their own lives and have a lot of other things to do. Even if we're lonely, we need to let go.
- We need to show our gratitude with hugs, kisses, and smiles. Expressions of joy and affirmation can go a long way toward making the caregiver feel important and appreciated. We're all doing the best we can.

Whether you are a caregiver or care receiver, it is best to try to see the dynamic from your partner's point of view. Tom, 67, strives to support his wife—his primary caregiver—as much as possible.

My wife helps take care of me. It has been very difficult for her. She feels wounded, too; we battle this disease together. I try to be as independent as I can, and I try not to take advantage of her. I give her time away from me and I try to make things as good for her as possible. That's my way of offering thanks.

Even with every attempt to respect your caregiver's needs, over time, your caregiver may still grow frustrated or overwhelmed by the challenge. Again, discuss the matter openly and try to come up with workable solutions rather than letting the resentment grow and fester. Untended, these negative feelings can turn into caregiver burnout.

▌ Caregiver Burnout

Caregiver burnout occurs when a caregiver feels emotionally, physically, and mentally exhausted; faced with ongoing responsibilities and limited energy, sometimes a caregiver can experience a change in attitude, either losing concern or feeling negatively toward the person with Parkinson's disease. Burnout threatens caregivers who feel unsupported or who can't keep up with the demands of the job. They may feel conflicted and guilty about their role, a situation that doesn't serve the caregiver or the care receiver.

The symptoms of burnout resemble those of depression. They include:

- ▌ Withdrawal
- ▌ Fatigue
- ▌ Anxiety
- ▌ Depression
- ▌ Feelings of hopelessness and helplessness
- ▌ Irritability
- ▌ Loss of interest in activities once enjoyed
- ▌ Changes in appetite, weight, or both
- ▌ Changes in sleep
- ▌ Getting sick more often
- ▌ Feelings of wanting to hurt yourself or person you are caring for
- ▌ Decrease in emotional and physical activities

Typically, burnout occurs when caregivers spend all their time caring for the person with Parkinson's and neglecting their own needs. Caring for a person with Parkinson's can be an unending and increasing task, and it can be confusing to work through your perceptions of your personal and caregiving roles. You may be a spouse, lover, child, friend, neighbor, or relative of a person with

Parkinson's, and you may feel some conflict about how those roles have changed. Too often caregivers feel it is their sole responsibility to support the care receiver, making it difficult to ask for help, especially in the times of greatest need.

Many caregivers feel frustrated that their efforts will not change the course of the disease. A gradual deterioration in abilities is expected over time; this is not a reflection of the quality of care a person with Parkinson's has received. Additional financial strains may further stress the household, especially if the spouse is also the caregiver.

To avoid burnout, you will probably need to ask for help both with the actual tasks involved with caregiving and with finding a safe place to talk about your feelings. For help with day-to-day assistance, ask friends for help, or contact a home-health nurse, adult day-care service provider, or short-term-care nurse. It is also essential that you find someone you can talk to about your frustrations. Caregiver support groups are available in many communities and online. Be open to talking about your feelings with a therapist, social worker, or member of the clergy if you feel burned out.

▌ Letter to My Friends and Family

The following letter, reprinted from an American Parkinson Disease Association newsletter, can be very helpful if you struggle to find the words to articulate your feelings to the people closest to you. I know many people who have copied this letter word for word and shared it with their loved ones.

> *I have Parkinson's disease. It is not catching or hereditary. No one knows what causes it, but some of the dopamine cells in the brain begin to die at an accelerated rate. Everyone slowly loses some dopamine cells as they grow older. If the*

cells suddenly begin to die at a faster rate, Parkinson's disease develops. It is slowly progressive and usually occurs as people get older. Medicine can help. I'll take newer, stronger kinds over the years. Some make me sick and take lots of adjustments. Stick with me. I have good days and bad days.

- *Tremors. You are expecting me to shake. Maybe I will, maybe I won't. Medicine today takes care of some of the tremors. If my hands, feet, or head are shaky, ignore it. I'll sit on my hand or put it in my pocket. Treat me as you always have. What is a little shakiness between friends?*

- *My face. You think you don't entertain me anymore because I'm not grinning or laughing. If I appear to stare at you or have a wooden expression, that's the Parkinson's. I hear you. I have the same intelligence. It just isn't as easy to show facial expression. If swallowing is a problem, I may drool. This bothers me, so we'll mop up.*

- *Stiffness. We are ready to go somewhere and as I get up, I can hardly move. Maybe my medicine is wearing off. This stiffness or rigidity is part of the Parkinson's. Let me take my time. Keep talking. I'll get there eventually. Trying to hurry me won't help. I can't hurry. I must take my time. If I seem jerky when I start out, that's normal. It will lessen as I get moving.*

- *Exercise. I need to walk every day. I will do as much as I can. Encourage me to go a little more each day. Walk with me. Company makes walking fun. It may be a slow walk but I'll get there. Remind me if I slump or stoop. I don't always know I'm doing this. My stretching, bending, pushing exercises must be done every day. Help with them if you can.*

- *My voice. As my deeper tones disappear, you'll notice*

my voice is getting higher and wispy. That's the Parkinson's. Listen to me. I know you can talk louder, faster, and finish my sentences for me. I hate that! Let me talk, get my thoughts together, and speak for myself. I'm still there. My mind is okay. Because I'm slower in movement, I talk more slowly too. I want to be part of the conversation. Let me speak.

- *Sleepiness. I may complain that I can't sleep. If I wander around in the middle of the night, that's the Parkinson's. It has nothing to do with what I ate or how early I went to bed. I may nap during the day. Let me sleep when I can. I can't always control when I'm tired or feel like sleeping.*

- *Emotions. Sometimes I cry and appear to be upset and you think you have done something to hurt my feelings. Probably not. It is the Parkinson's. Keep talking to me. Ignore the tears. I'll be okay in a few minutes.*

Patience, my friend. I need you. I'm the same person, I've just slowed down. It's not easy to talk about Parkinson's, but I'll try if you want me to. I need my friends. I want to continue to be part of life. Please remain my friend.

I do not know who wrote this, but I know I sent it to my family and friends and got a great response. It helped them know and maybe understand what a day with Parkinson's disease is like for us.

▮ Accepting Change

While the role of caregiver can be an exhausting and at times frustrating one, it can also be infinitely rewarding. Many people do not allow themselves to open up emotionally until they face a serious crisis. Parkinson's disease will inevitably alter the balance of many relationships, including the bond between the caregiver and care receiver, and this change can present an opportunity for both parties to grow closer and more appreciative of what they can learn from one another. For most of us, this journey isn't easy, simple, or straight; it will almost certainly require a lot of conscious effort on the part of the caregiver and the person with Parkinson's so that they can both understand the many ways the relationship has changed.

People with Parkinson's who are also caregivers for another person must accept the changes in their relationships as both caregivers and receivers. For some it can be very frustrating; Carol, 63, has had Parkinson's since she was 49, but she also helps to care for her elderly mother.

"My mom isn't well. She's 88, and I need to help take care of her, but I can't," says Carol. "One night I was alone with her and I needed to put a diaper on her. I stayed up all night trying, but I just couldn't do it. It bothers me. I want to be able to take care of my mom, but I can't."

Carol has had to accept her limitations and care for her mother in other ways. Some days she can do more of the physical work; other days she can't really take care of herself. This is the nature of Parkinson's, and, unfortunately, we have to live by the rules of the disease. Carol does a great deal for her mother, and she's doing the best she can. What more can anyone ask? We all need to learn to be compassionate with ourselves.

Part 4 of this book explores surviving and thriving with Parkinson's disease. People with Parkinson's continually discover new ways of working around our symptoms to normalize our days. Chapter 14 shares some of the approaches that others have found useful.

PART FOUR

Surviving and Thriving with Parkinson's Disease

14

Practical Suggestions for Facing Daily Challenges

A few years ago, Michael attended a formal dinner for a political candidate he supported. He tried to cut his meat, but the harder he tried, the more he floundered. Embarrassed, the candidate himself offered to help Michael with his food. "I was tired of knocking my food on the floor," Michael said. "I vowed to find a way to be independent."

The solution? Michael decided to cut his meat with a sharp pair of scissors. "It was a discovery borne of desperation and hunger," Michael joked. "But it works."

It's a marvelous solution. By pinning the food to the plate with the tip of the shears and snipping, almost anyone with Parkinson's can manage to cut with independence and dignity. (It's particularly easy with spring-loaded shears that open upon release.) Until Michael came up with this inspired idea, we threw a lot of food on the floor and lived by the 30-second rule—food on the floor less than 30 seconds is safe to eat. I now keep a pair of scissors in my purse all the time.

For the most part, discoveries like this come from trial and error. This chapter lists many practical suggestions for ways you can make your life easier or more efficient. Some of these solutions may help to minimize or eliminate some of the challenges you may face every day.

▮ Food and Medication

▮ Take a sip of soda before taking your medication. The soda coats the stomach, minimizing side effects. (If you find that you need to use milk instead, only drink enough to get the medication down; the protein in the milk can cause your medication to be less effective.)

▮ Avoid eating protein within one or two hours of taking levodopa. Many people avoid this problem by eating fruit in the morning, vegetables at lunch, and protein (meat, fish, eggs, cheese) at dinner. However, I would recommend that you consume carbohydrates at dinner for energy; we have enough problems with low energy without cutting carbs.

▮ Always carry extra medication when you're out for the day. You never know if you're going to need it. I carry a bag of medication everywhere I go.

▮ Take along a bottle of water to combat dry mouth and to help swallow pills. If your medication makes you nauseous, bring along a few crackers to absorb the excess stomach acid caused by the medication.

▮ Drink from a straw. People with Parkinson's sometimes find it difficult to drink from a glass without tremors and spills. On formal occasions, I carry a decorated straw.

▮ Ask for a chair with arms when dining out. You may find that you have more control over your hands if you can rest your arms. In addition, the arms on the chair will make it much easier to stand up at the end of the meal.

▮ Trade your fork for a spoon. Many people with Parkinson's find it easier to manipulate a spoon than a fork. I am forever dropping food right in the middle of my shirt because my tremors make food drip off the end of my fork.

▌ Don't rush your meal. It may take you longer than someone without Parkinson's to finish your dinner, but don't hurry. Instead, relax and enjoy some meaningful conversation.

▌ There may be times when it's easier to use your fingers than your utensils. Don't feel embarrassed, just enjoy your meal.

▌ Ask for a private table if you think your tremors or habits will distract other diners. You may feel more comfortable in a secluded setting.

▌ Gadgets

▌ Use an electric razor. Many models are easy to grip, and you can eliminate the need to struggle with small, sharp blade razors.

▌ Switch to an electric toothbrush with a large handle for easy grip. If tremors are a problem in putting toothpaste on the brush, try placing it in your hand or on your finger. (Make sure you put the brush in your mouth before turning it on or the toothpaste goes all over the room—learn from my mistake.)

▌ Buy a one-handed can opener.

▌ Wear your keys on a large strap around your neck to minimize fumbling with them.

▌ Install grab bars in the showers and along hallways.

▌ Buy a walker so you have it when you need it.

▌ Install an elevated toilet seat. It will be easier to stand if you are not crouched down as far.

▌ Use a handheld showerhead to minimize falls in the shower. If necessary, sit on a shower seat while showering.

▌ Use soap on a rope to minimize scrambling for runaway soap while bathing.

- To make it easier to turn over in bed, try sheets made of satin or nylon.
- Tie a knotted rope onto the corner of the bed so that you can pull yourself over using your arms.
- Wear slip-on shoes and use a shoehorn. You may want to try some clothing with Velcro closures.

■ Preventing Falls

People with Parkinson's are most vulnerable to falls when they are getting up from a chair, sitting down in a chair, turning while walking, stepping off or onto a curb, and taking the first few steps when walking. To prevent falls:

- Use a walker. Some people prefer walkers with wheels; others find that wheeled walkers can slip away from them too quickly, actually causing falls. If you have a wheeled walker that moves too quickly, remove the wheels and replace them with tennis balls that allow you to push the walker in a slower, more controlled movement. You may also want to consider a wheeled walker with hand brakes and a seat.
- Carry a cane, either a standard one or a quad (a cane with four legs that can stand unsupported). At age 40, I use a cane, but I decorate it so I look stylish. Don't hesitate to use a cane out of pride; you'll look much better walking with a cane than falling without one.
- Avoid high-heeled shoes.
- If you shuffle when you walk, replace your rubber-soled shoes with leather-soled footwear.
- Work with a physical therapist to use your arms and take wider steps to improve your balance.
- Treadmill walking, yoga, and tai chi can strengthen the muscles and improve balance, reducing your risk of falling.

▌ Remove throw rugs and electric wires from the floor to minimize tripping hazards.

▌ Sit on the bed or a chair when dressing and undressing.

▌ Consciously think about each movement before you do it. Re-
hearse it in your mind's eye before you start moving.

▌ Freeze Attacks

About 30 percent of people with Parkinson's experience freezing,
temporarily losing the ability to move. The problem is more common among people who have problems with walking and balance.
Freezing occurs most often when getting up from a chair or bed,
walking through a doorway, entering tight spaces or an elevator,
climbing stairs, and turning corners.

Here are some tricks that may help you break a freeze.

▌ Imagine a line on the floor and try to step over it. (If it helps,
you may want to put tape on the floor near doorways preced-
ing turns to give you something to step over.)

▌ Imagine marching in formation and then step out and begin to
march across the floor.

▌ Take aim and step toward a specific tile or mark on the floor.

▌ If someone is with you, ask him to put his foot out so you
have something to step over.

▌ Rock from side to side to build momentum for the first step.

▌ Use a cane equipped with a plastic attachment that gives you
something to step over.

▌ Try a cane equipped with a laser pointer that projects a line to
step over similar to the plastic attachment.

▌ Trained companion dogs assist some people with Parkinson's
in recovering from a freeze. These dogs can be trained to tap
a person's foot with their paws; these dogs also help with balance and with getting up after a fall. Studies have found that

well-trained dogs can reduce the risk of falls by 75 to 80 percent.

▮ Don't rely on a walker if you're prone to freeze attacks. Researchers have found that people with Parkinson's who use walkers (both standard and wheeled designs) freeze more often than those who walked on their own.

▮ Speaking and Swallowing Problems

▮ Work on speaking problems as soon as they appear. Consult a speech therapist for exercises to deal with slurring or a weak voice. (Once you experience significant changes in your speech, it is much more difficult to reverse the situation.) In most cases, speech therapy involves both breathing and tongue, lip, and jaw exercises.

▮ Take a deep breath before speaking. Use short sentences with frequent pauses to keep your volume strong.

▮ Ask your doctor about collagen injections if your speech problems are caused by vocal cord weakness. In this treatment, collagen is injected into the vocal cords, increasing their size and making them more effective at making sound.

▮ Vocal cord implants are another option when someone has lost the ability to speak completely.

▮ Handheld microphones and other amplification devices are nonsurgical alternatives.

▮ Writing Problems

▮ If you have difficulty writing, try "fat" pens with special grips that make them easier to hold. Similarly, you can put a rubber band around a pen you already have to make it fatter and easier to grasp.

▌ If you have trouble signing your name, ask your bank to make a signature stamp that can be used in place of your legal signature.

▌ Use your computer or typewriter to assist with some writing tasks, if it is easier. Voice-activated computer software can make it easier for some people to communicate without typing at all.

▌ Going Out

It is vital that people with Parkinson's get out and interact with the world, rather than pulling in and isolating ourselves. We must find ways to make our trips easier, whether we're traveling across town or across the country.

▌ Use an electric scooter if having one makes you willing to get out and visit the mall or grocery store. I use them and typically have a more enjoyable time than I do when I'm stubborn—and ultimately exhausted—by walking everywhere on my own.

▌ At a buffet restaurant, put your personal belongings at the table and then ask someone to go with you to fill and carry your plate as you point out what you want.

▌ If you are shopping alone, don't hesitate to ask for help in transporting your purchases to your car.

▌ On a long drive, take a standard pillow or neck pillow with you to rest.

▌ Make sure your medication and a bottle of water are handy in the car.

▌ Take it easy when you travel. If you're tired or stiff, take a break. Michael and I have pushed to get where we're going, only to find we've overdone it and we're so exhausted the next day we can't enjoy the trip.

▌ When flying, make arrangements for handicapped assistance when you buy your ticket. Even if you feel you can walk in the terminal, you're better off with help. In airports, people are in a hurry and bags clutter the ground, increasing the risk of falling. Having assistance when boarding can often ease the burden on your travel partner as well.

▌ Make sure to take your medication with you in your carry-on baggage so you'll have it if you need it. I usually have backup meds in my checked baggage as well, in case my carry-on bag is lost or stolen.

▌ At hotels, ask for extra pillows if you need them to get comfortable.

▌ Ask for a first-floor room when staying at a hotel. You should also check the location of emergency exits. If you need to evacuate the building during an emergency, you want to know where you are going and be able to avoid stairs.

▌ If you order room service, consider asking to have the meat cut for you in the kitchen.

General Information

▌ Prepare a packet of information about Parkinson's disease, your medications, and any other medical history that might be useful to someone taking care of you. I carry a notebook which I call my PD Bible. It lists pages of personal and medical information, including two summary pages titled "What Is PD?" and "How to Treat Me." I include these pages because I have some unique health issues, such as orthostatic hypotension, and I do not always run a fever with an infection, so it is vital that medical staff who might treat me in an emergency room or hospital have this information.

▌ Take all relevant information with you if you go to the emergency room and when you travel.

▌ If you are traveling alone, consider giving an information sheet about PD to the hotel manager. If you're staying with a friend who doesn't know much about the disease, you might want to provide information about PD. Information goes a long way toward making other people feel comfortable.

▌ The Benefits of Physical Therapy

Don't disregard the importance of physical and occupational therapy, offered at hospitals, medical centers, or through many visiting nurses. Many of the techniques you learn will help you maintain your flexibility and independence as long as possible.

For many people with Parkinson's disease, the treatment involves learning "movement strategies"—ways to roll over in bed, get up from a chair, or climb out of a car. A therapist may tell you about simple devices to assist with day-to-day activities and allow you to maintain your independence and dignity. Don't delay asking for help; there's a lot we can learn from each other. Some reliable companies that specialize in products designed for people with Parkinson's follow:

Clothing and Assistive Devices List

Planet Amber
www.planetamber.com

Sammons Preston
(800) 323-5547
www.sammonspreston.com

Wardrobe Wagon
(800) 992-2737
www.wardrobewagon.com

Bruce Medical Supply
(800) 225-8446
www.brucemedical.com

While these tips can help you overcome the physical challenges of living with Parkinson's, you will also need to focus on a number of emotional challenges associated with the disease. In addition to learning new ways of dressing yourself and cutting your food, you will also need to learn to accept help from other people. For some of us, that isn't easy. Over time, your relationships will change—you won't be able to do the things you once did and you will discover new strengths and skills you may never have imagined. Chapter 15 explores some of the ways your relationships with your family and friends will change and how you can allow your Parkinson's disease to refocus and strengthen your relationships with those closest to you.

15

Parkinson's Disease Touches Everyone: Working Through Changes in Your Relationships

There's no getting around the simple truth: Parkinson's disease will change every relationship you have—with your spouse, your dependent children, your grown children, your parents, your friends, your extended family, your coworkers, even strangers you encounter in the checkout line at the grocery store. Like it or not, people will see you in a different light; they will treat you differently. Some people will feel uncomfortable and pull away; others will prove their dedication to you and stand with you on some of the darkest nights. Some people will hurt your feelings; others will make you feel more blessed than you ever imagined possible.

The emotional side of Parkinson's disease should begin to be addressed as soon as someone is diagnosed with the disease. The early weeks after diagnosis can be a very lonely and difficult time, and often those closest to you aren't sure how to react or what to say. Often people mean well but end up making remarks that only make you feel worse. At the time I learned of my Parkinson's, I lived in a small town and the members of my church and people who knew me casually often greeted me with comments such as, "Great to see you. Are you feeling better?" They were simply uninformed—they didn't understand that I had a progressive, degenerative disease and would not get better—but their words stung because they reminded me that I was not ever going to be the same person I was before this disease invaded my life.

People closest to me often turned to me, asking me what was going to happen next. They wanted to know what the future would hold, how this disease would change us. Again and again I had to say, "I don't know." Many people with Parkinson's find that they are struggling to make sense of everything that is happening to their bodies at the same time that their partners and family members are trying to make sense of what changes are happening in their relationships. Frankly, those of us with Parkinson's can't make sense of the future when we can barely meet the challenges of the day ahead. It takes a while to accept the diagnosis and settle into the realities of life with Parkinson's.

It may come as no surprise that many people with Parkinson's end up divorced within a few years of their diagnosis. Both Michael and I had marriages that ended in divorce under the strain of our diagnoses; those couples I know who have been able to stay together have done so because they work tirelessly on building and maintaining communication with their spouses. Marriage isn't easy under the best of circumstances, and it is that much more difficult with the added burden of living with Parkinson's.

This chapter will explore the dynamics associated with many types of relationships and how they may change after the diagnosis of Parkinson's disease.

∎ Seeing Parkinson's from the Other's Point of View

Parkinson's disease affects everyone around us. We may feel the painful realities of Parkinson's every day, but our loved ones must live with the disease, too. Ideally, family and close friends should become informed about the disease so that they can understand what is happening—and will happen—to our bodies. The more they know about the illness, the better equipped they will be to handle the physical and emotional challenges.

Unfortunately, those closest to us can sometimes be unable to appreciate our struggles. In some cases, people close to those with Parkinson's can experience denial; they simply don't accept that you have the disease and that your condition is going to decline. They may blame us if we have energy to go shopping in the morning but feel too exhausted to go out to dinner by late afternoon. Children may not accept that we can't gather the strength to attend a ball game or school play when we were once our child's number one booster. Even if they want to understand, they can't comprehend the toll the disease takes on our bodies, minds, and emotions; no matter what we describe or tell them, they can't feel it.

"My husband was heartbroken when I was diagnosed," said Marian, who was diagnosed at age 52, "but he didn't know what he was heartbroken about. I gave him literature about the disease, but he didn't want to read it. He was afraid to know. I'm the one living with it, but he's the one having the hard time."

The most meaningful thing we can do to overcome this obstacle is to communicate—both to listen and to share our feelings. We need to talk, we need to listen; we need to ask questions, we need to be open to hearing answers that may make us uncomfortable.

In addition, our attitude plays a critical role in guiding our relationships. How we discuss the disease and talk about our experiences will have a major impact on the tone of conversation. We must genuinely believe that we are not our disease—I am still the same Gretchen I have always been, although I now have Parkinson's disease—and in the future I will continue to love and share with the people I love. While my daughter was growing up, I may not have been able to make it to every one of her horse shows, but

I'd like to think I found other ways to express my love for her and support her interests.

Having a healthy attitude about our illness and future is our responsibility; we cannot expect our partners or caregivers to make us feel good about our lives. Of course, early in the disease you may be reeling from the diagnosis and not ready to embrace the future, but for your own sake, you will need to do whatever is necessary to reclaim your optimism and accept your destiny.

Michael and I are our own support team, and we do, of course, experience days of desperation. We have an agreement, however: We allow ourselves brief pity parties, when we indulge every bit of unhappy, why-me, it's-not-fair attitude. After about 15 minutes, the one who isn't feeling so blue pops the balloons and declares that the party is over: Now, what are you going to do about your problem? (We also have an agreement that only one of us can feel self-pitying at a time.)

This approach involves communication—of both the feelings of frustration and loss and the feelings of concern and the desire to take action. Relationships that do not have strong communication skills before the time of diagnosis may benefit from professional counseling to open the lines of communication before resentments and miscommunications take their toll.

▌ Relationships with Spouses

Inevitably, Parkinson's disease will change the balance of your relationship. Your partner will have a number of questions: How is this disease going to affect you? How will it affect me? What are you going to be able to bring to me in this relationship? What am I going to need to do for you?

If you are married, you and your partner vowed to love one another in times of sickness and health, but realistically the demands of living with a chronic, debilitating illness can overwhelm many people. The relationships of people with young-onset Parkinson's face the special challenge of dealing with decades of caregiving and diminishing capacity; someone who married expecting to live into old age with a healthy partner may not be able to imagine becoming a caregiver to a spouse who needs assistance at age 34. The healthy partner may also be left with the added burden of working longer hours to pay the bills and caring for young children who may not get all the attention they need from the partner with Parkinson's.

My marriage lasted 11 years and Michael's 12 years before they crumbled under the difficult realities of Parkinson's disease. We have known people in 25-year marriages that couldn't survive the stress. Michael's wife told him it was like having the rug pulled out from under her; it was too much reality too fast. My husband did the best he could at the time to accept my illness, but in the end our marriage felt like a union of obligation and neither of us was happy.

That said, we also know people whose marriages have grown stronger because both partners dedicate themselves to combating the disease together. Kellie, 37, went through DBS surgery with her husband of 20 years at her side. "The night before my brain surgery, my husband and I both shaved our heads," she said. "People said, 'You two look alike.' My husband was with me every step of the way."

Just as Michael and I take turns being strong, in these relationships both the person with Parkinson's and the spouse-caregiver take turns being strong. Both parties tend to appreciate and try to understand the struggles faced by the other partner. It isn't easy living with Parkinson's disease, whether you're the person with the disease or the person loving and caring for the person with the disease.

In many cases, the healthy partner feels some guilt at the time of diagnosis in response to harsh comments that may have been made about the person with Parkinson's. By the time we learn we have Parkinson's, many of us have spent years feeling tired, stumbling, experiencing sexual dysfunction, and other problems; since these symptoms weren't associated with a disease, our partner may have blamed us for being lazy, aloof, cold, or withdrawn from the relationship. When they learn about the illness, they may feel guilty about feeling these things and say, "I'm so sorry about all the cruel things I said; I didn't realize you were really sick."

The only way to get through this process and to build a healthy new relationship is to communicate clearly and compassionately about everything you are both going through. Together, you and your partner need to learn about the disease, talk about the disease, and talk about your relationship and what you can and cannot do for each other. Many relationships thrive under the support of a marriage counselor who can help a couple build the necessary communication skills, as well as the ongoing support offered by Parkinson's support groups for people with Parkinson's and their caregivers.

Gary, 50, believes a lack of communication undermined his marriage. "One of the problems with couples is that neither partner really knows what's going on," he said. "Both parties feel insecurity and fear about what the future holds, but most people have trouble talking about it. I don't know anyone who hasn't had problems with communication.

"One thing that is lacking is counseling about what to expect," said Gary, who was divorced two years after he learned he had PD. "I think part of the diagnosis should be an explanation of how this disease will affect your life and relationships. The psychological aspects can be more devastating than the physical symptoms. I don't know whether counseling could have saved my marriage, but I do know that the psychological pressure was the straw that broke the camel's back."

▌ Relationships with Dependent Children

When you talk about Parkinson's disease with your young children, the fist thing you need to do is assure them that you're not going to die. Very young children don't understand death, but by elementary school, most children fear it, even if they don't completely understand it. All children need reassurance that while you may reach a point when you will not be able to attend all of their activities or play catch in the backyard, you will always love them and be with them as best you can.

"When we told the kids, they were devastated," said Karen R., who was diagnosed at age 44. "They thought I was going to die. I told them Parkinson's wouldn't kill me. I said I would be there to dance at their weddings—but I might not be able to dance too long." Over time, the children, both in high school, came to accept the situation.

"Once they realized I wasn't going to die, they didn't want to know anything about what was happening with me," Karen said. "One day I asked my daughter to bring up the laundry basket. She was perturbed. I thought, 'If you aren't willing to do the little things for me, how are you going to help with the big things?' It was difficult for her to understand that I needed some help."

Ironically, the younger the child, the more accepting he or she can be about Parkinson's. These kids live with you and all of the shaking and freezing; they may not remember a time when you didn't have tremors. When Michael's son introduces his father to a new friend, he says, "This is my dad. He has Parkinson's, so don't worry if he shakes and twitches"—then he runs off to play.

Marian, 60, has five children, eleven grandchildren, and one great-grandchild. "My grandchildren are much more accepting and sympathetic than my children because the only way they know me is with Parkinson's," she said. "My children have trouble because I'm not the same person I once was and they feel they have lost someone."

In addition, older dependent kids may feel angry about the limitations on your time and energy. They may remember when you were able to offer them more attention and participate in their lives more fully, and they may resent both you and the illness for cutting into what they feel entitled to receive from you. In addition, teenagers may feel embarrassed by your symptoms; at an age when every teenager is humiliated to be seen with his or her parents, it can be that much more difficult to be seen with parents who actually do look and act different in public.

"I used to coach my son's T-ball team and my daughter's basketball team," said Boyd, who was diagnosed at age 44. "It became more and more difficult, and I had to give it up. My kids tell me they miss their father; they want their old dad back. I tell them I understand—I wish for that, too."

Again, the importance of attitude comes into play. You may not be able to do everything you once did, but your kids need to see you living your life. They need to see you participating in life as much as you can and in whatever ways you find possible. You can teach your children a great deal about the values of perseverance and optimism by making the most you can with what you have been given. You can inspire your children to realize their God-given potential because your life is an example of fulfilling your own destiny with joy and celebration.

My Parkinson's symptoms were in full bloom when my daughter was a "tween," an almost-teenager. At that time, having a mother with one hair out of place was embarrassing, having a mother who walked with a cane or used a scooter in the grocery store was mortifying. At that time, I didn't have a very positive attitude; I wasn't sure how I felt about this disease, but I knew I was afraid and resentful. I keenly felt all that I had lost, and did not fully appreciate all that I had left. Still, I did my best to reassure my daughter that we were okay; we were a family; we would survive.

My daughter just wanted her old mom back. She never wanted to talk about the Parkinson's. I think she felt that if we didn't talk about it, we could deny the disease was there and turn back the clock. I continued to try to get her to talk about her feelings, and as time went on, she gradually began to open up. Today, she tells me how proud she is of me and the work I do. She's told me she's blessed to have me as a mom. I feel truly blessed that we reached this level of awareness, but it took a long time for both of us to make peace with the situation and build a new relationship.

Jeremy, who was diagnosed with PD at age 30, has enough faith in his future that he and his wife decided to have a child. "My wife has been here for me, and she's very supportive of everything," he said. "My son is now five months old. My ongoing prayer was that he wouldn't be born with problems. He is fine, and that has been my greatest blessing."

The process of living with Parkinson's has changed Jeremy's outlook on other issues as well. "I am much more humble and accepting of others than I used to be," he said. "I'm a lot nicer and more polite. I had a wake-up call. Sometimes when people get on my nerves, I accept the situation. I try to let the anger pass through me so that I can see the good in people. I think that makes me a better father to my son."

▌ Relationships with Grown Children

Adult children with parents who are in their seventies at the time of diagnosis may not have difficulty accepting the diagnosis; they expected their parents to develop some health challenges as they grew older. Those young adults whose parents may be in their forties or fifties when diagnosed may feel a greater burden since they may feel the need to care for their parents while meeting the demands of young children, high-pressure jobs, and other commitments. They may still be trying to get their own lives together and be less willing to accept that their parents may need help earlier than they expected.

Once again, communication and attitude will determine how the situation evolves. If we can remain positive and see the situation from all points of view, the more likely those around us will be able to do the same. Try to acknowledge and accept the demands on the lives of your children and take these factors into account when determining how to ask for help. Keep them informed of your health decisions and let them know what they can do to help you. Be sure to openly discuss what you need from them, so that you won't feel resentment about what they are not doing for you and they won't feel resentment about you asking for help when they already feel their lives are busy enough. Bottom line: Talk through the situation and set clear expectations about how both you and your children can create clear boundaries that allow both sides to offer support and concern that do not feel like an undue burden.

▌ Relationships with Parents

The relationship between a person with Parkinson's and his or her parents can be tricky. Parents sometimes feel guilty and blame themselves: Was the disease caused by something I did? Something I didn't do? Sometimes parents try to deny the illness, feeling that in the natural order of things the child is supposed to be healthy and care for the parents during their golden years. In addition, some parents may feel that once their children are grown, their role as primary caregiver is over and they can claim more time for themselves. They may feel somewhat cheated by the reality that they may need to continue to help their child on an ongoing basis.

The person with Parkinson's may feel guilty about not being able to care for his or her parents as they age. Those of us who are younger and have parents in their seventies and eighties wish that we could stand up and help our parents out, but too often we can't stand at all. We have to lean on our parents more than we want to; in this relationship we want to be the caregivers rather than care receivers, but we can't be.

Michael, a 48-year-old who was diagnosed at age 35, has had to ask his parents for help. "My parents have seen me deteriorate over the years. When I was freezing a lot, I once got stuck in the bathroom and I couldn't get out for an hour and a half. I had to holler for my dad to come and get me, then I had to crawl from the bathroom to the bedroom. I knew if I tried to walk, I'd fall. My dad has sacrificed so much to help me, and it's been hard on all of us."

I am grateful that my mom is a strong, vibrant 67-year-old, but I worry about what might happen if she gets sick. I want to tell her, "Sit down and I'll take care of you," but too often I'm the one who needs help.

To minimize the potential for conflict, we must keep our parents in the loop. We need to openly discuss with them what we need and what we wish we could do for them. The more we can find ways to communicate about the disease, the better off we will all be. The better informed our parents are, the less frightened they will be; the more knowledgeable they become, the closer these relationships will be.

▌ Relationships with Siblings

The kind of conversation you might have with your brothers and sisters about Parkinson's disease probably depends on the closeness of the relationship before the diagnosis. Siblings may find the news somewhat personally threatening, especially if you have any reason to believe that your sibling shared any kind of toxic environmental exposures when you where children. The genetic risk of Parkinson's is described in Chapter 2; you may want to review this material and talk it over with your siblings when you talk about the disease.

Michael's sister, Wendy, provided tremendous assistance to him and encouraged him to join a support group; his brother, Rick, has become a Parkinson's advocate in Maryland. In many ways, the disease has brought Michael closer to some family members, joining the family together in the shared mission of overcoming Parkinson's.

My two sisters have not been as active, but they have always been supportive. My older sister, Carol, and my younger sister, Carrie, stay current on PD issues and offer to help me in any way possible. Their support in the battle against Parkinson's on my behalf has made me feel appreciated and loved.

▮ Relationships with Friends

When you're diagnosed with Parkinson's disease, you find out who your real friends are. Some people pull away; others come much closer. I've had both types of friends. When I was first diagnosed I don't know how I could have made it without my dear friend Jess. She took me to doctor's appointments; she picked up the slack in our relationship without my saying anything. Sometimes she would listen while I tried to make sense of what was happening to me, and at other times she sat quietly and I felt comfort in the silence. There were times when I actually fell asleep in the middle of a sentence, and she let me doze off and then reminded me of what I was talking about when I woke up a few minutes later. I couldn't have asked any more from her.

Other people avoided me because they didn't know how to deal with me. They were suddenly unavailable, and they didn't return phone calls. I felt like a leper, at a time when I really needed to be around other people. Michael had the same experience, especially with his friends in politics. Because of his outward symptoms, he became politically embarrassing—would people think he was drunk or using drugs? Was he simply strange? Michael learned just how shallow some of those people were, and it was a difficult time for him.

Ultimately, we must all accept our disease and give other people the opportunity to do so as well. If those around us don't want to become better informed and can't get past the outward symptoms of the disease, there is nothing we can do to make them accept us. In these cases, I have found it best to accept that the friendship is ending because the other person can't make room in the relationship for the Parkinson's disease and move forward. While this feels like a personal rejection, it's really not about you at all. Some people simply don't feel comfortable dealing with serious issues of illness and disease, and they can't maintain the friendship any longer.

Now many of our friends have only known us as people with Parkinson's, and some of our closest friends actually forget that we have the disease. There are times when we're with a group and we become tired and need to rest, and we actually have to remind them that we need to slow down because of the Parkinson's. We consider this a great compliment; we are accepted as peers first and people with Parkinson's second. When this happens, we know we're really living.

One of the challenges of accepting Parkinson's involves maintaining the quality of our relationships once the diagnosis becomes public. "As soon as they knew, all my friends started treating me differently," said Karen R. "I'd pull up in the driveway for a picnic, and everyone would rush up and say, 'Are you feeling okay?' 'Do you want me to help carry anything?' I'm still the same person; if I need help, I'll ask." It can be difficult to protect your independence from well-intentioned friends who want to help—a bit too much. It's best, once again, to clearly communicate your feelings: "I appreciate your concern, but it isn't necessary. Please know that I will ask for help if I need it."

▮ Relationships with Strangers

Although we don't always think of it as such, we have relationships with the strangers we encounter from day to day. Since these people don't know us at all, they are responding to our outward appearance and behavior—and trust me, that can lead to lots of misunderstanding. Often when I go into a convenience store, people look at me as if I'm a drug addict in need of a trip to a methadone clinic. Or they think I'm mentally challenged. On the other hand, some strangers will respond by going out of their way to be helpful and hold the door open for me or offer to reach at item placed on an upper shelf. I think people's behavior during these casual encounters reveals a lot about them.

When I'm out in public, I feel invisible and too visible at the same time. Sometimes I feel that every tremor or stumble makes me stand out in the crowd, while at other times people try so hard to ignore me that they literally walk right into me. I've lost count of how often people have kicked my cane out from under me or crashed into my scooter while they were preoccupied with not noticing my handicap. They're typically apologetic and embarrassed, but they don't usually treat me like just another person in the store.

Most of the time I don't bother trying to explain that I have Parkinson's to the people I meet. Occasionally I do encounter someone who recognizes what he or she is looking at because they have a family member or friend with the disease; sometimes a person might make a remark about Parkinson's disease, but typically it goes unspoken. Since Michael J. Fox has made Parkinson's disease a more public illness, more people have a general understanding of the disease and seem to be more willing to talk about it.

▌ The Five Be's of Relationships

In any relationship, even one untouched by Parkinson's disease, communication is essential. The more open and honest you are and the more information you share, the greater the possibility of closeness. The only way others can understand what you're feeling and going through is if you tell them. You need to share the good feelings and the bad.

In essence, building and maintaining strong relationships comes down to five critical "Be's."

▌ *Be educated.* You need to learn as much as possible about Parkinson's disease, and you need to share that information with your family and friends. They need to understand the disease so that they can understand how it is challenging you.

▌ *Be open and honest.* Honest, direct communication isn't easy, but it is essential if you want to avoid misunderstandings and resentments. You need to acknowledge the conflicts and confusing feelings your loved ones may experience, and you should be willing to allow them the freedom to feel overwhelmed by your diagnosis. Parkinson's disease touches the entire family.

▌ *Be positive.* In most cases, your loved ones will take the lead from you. The more optimistic you can be, the more optimistic they will be.

▌ *Be patient*—with yourself and with the others around you. Realize that dealing with PD will take more than a single heart-to-heart conversation that magically clears emotions forever. All relationships evolve over time, and it is especially the case now. You're going to have some ups and downs; accept them and allow your relationships to change and grow over time.

▌ *Be willing to ask for help.* When communication breaks down and all else fails, you may benefit from meeting with a third party or mediator. This person could be another caregiver, a friend, a member of the clergy, or a therapist. The presence of a different point of view can sometimes lend clarity and a new perspective to the dynamic. If the relationship is in trouble or in emotional turbulence, seek professional counseling.

In addition to the inevitable changes in your personal relationships, Parkinson's disease will also force you to wrestle with practical concerns about securing your financial future. Chapter 16 looks at how to handle workplace challenges, disability, and Social Security.

16

Financial Challenges: Facing Job Loss, Disability, Social Security, and Insurance Struggles

I was devastated when my Parkinson's symptoms became bad enough that I had to give up my job. I had worked as an autism specialist and early-childhood educator for 18 years. When I had to give up my career, I felt that part of me was dying. Parkinson's was forcing me to become someone new, whether I wanted to or not.

At first, I scaled back to three-quarter time. My employer was very gracious in allowing me to do so. My sleep patterns were so disrupted, I would come in three days at noon and two days full-time. At lunch hour I went into the physical therapy room and napped. I couldn't make it through the day without a break.

When I had to quit my job, I had trouble getting disability because of my age. It took more than two and a half years to get my benefits approved. During that time, I had no income. I am divorced now, but when I was going through this period I was married; my husband and I had to declare bankruptcy. We spent both my retirement and my husband's retirement savings just to make ends meet.

In the end, my case was heard by a judge. At the time, no one from Social Security had ever met me; all they knew about me came from the papers I filled out. On the record, the judge apologized to me, noting that I had given my life to the betterment of our society's children and that I should have been treated fairly. He told the attorney from the Social Security Administration that it was not right that I had been physically devastated by the disease and then financially devastated by the government. I felt vindicated and my case was approved, but I still felt like I had barely survived a nightmare.

Unfortunately, my situation is all too common. In this chapter, we will discuss the financial challenges faced by someone with Parkinson's disease, including job loss, Social Security Disability benefits, and health insurance. In addition to the physical and emotional toll this disease takes on someone with Parkinson's, it can be financially crippling as well.

▌ Job Loss: Talking to Your Employer

For each of us the timing may be different, but sooner or later we will all have to discuss our Parkinson's disease with our employers. Some people can go for years with only mild symptoms or symptoms completely controlled with medication, while others may experience a faster progression of the disease. For each of us, however, there is a line that we will cross when we can no longer do the work we once performed with ease.

Each employment scenario needs to be assessed individually. In general terms, I recommend that you discuss the situation with your boss at the time the disease begins to interfere with your job performance. You don't want to have to overcome a poor performance evaluation; your employer may dismiss the Parkinson's diagnosis as an excuse for not doing your best. If you need to miss a meeting because of a doctor's appointment or if you simply can't keep up the pace you once did, you want your boss to know that the Parkinson's is to blame.

Your boss and coworkers may notice changes in your behavior long before you think they will. If you tend to have tremors or balance problems or slurred speech, your employer may assume you have an alcohol or drug problem rather than Parkinson's disease.

Kellie, who was diagnosed at age 32, worked in a medical office. "About a year after I was diagnosed, I started to slow down," she said. "My boss really tormented me over it. She said I couldn't have Parkinson's because nobody my age has it. She kept writing me up, ultimately forcing me to quit my job."

If possible, try to approach your boss—or a higher-level supervisor, if necessary—before you develop serious problems at work. When speaking to your employer, approach the situation with a positive attitude. Let your employer know what you *can* do and how you can maintain performance with medication. In some cases, you may be able to adjust your hours or telecommute to extend your period of employment as long as possible. Before you begin to negotiate with your employer, review the company sick policy and health insurance plans so you know what benefits you're entitled to.

In theory, the Americans with Disabilities Act (ADA) should protect you from discrimination at work, but in the real world, things don't always work out as intended. I know lots of people who have been fired from their jobs because of their PD. If an employer wants to get rid of you, he or she is going to find a way to do it, by documenting poor performance or taking the chance that you won't appeal the decision. When you go in to speak to your boss, don't say, "The ADA says you have to make special accommodations for me," which can set a negative tone, as if you're trying to pick a fight. Try to make specific suggestions and design a plan for follow-up.

When you first speak to your employer, you may just want to share the information, rather than ask for accommodations to do your job. If your symptoms have reached the point where you need to make changes in your work arrangements, try to be as specific as possible about what you need and how the changes will allow you to continue in your job. In other words, try to suggest solutions, rather than simply stating the problems.

After meeting with your boss, ask for a written summary of your conversation and any agreements. This paper trail may be very important if you need to document your history of disability for any reason.

▮ Disability Programs

If you lose your job because you are disabled by your Parkinson's symptoms, you may qualify for benefits. There are a number of disability programs, but the primary ones are Social Security Disability Insurance (SSDI), Supplemental Security Income (SSI), Medicare, State Health Insurance Counseling and Assistance Programs (SHIP), and Medicaid. In addition, some employers offer private disability insurance as part of their benefits package.

From the time you are diagnosed with Parkinson's, it is essential that you get a big box or set up a filing system and save every scrap of paper you receive about your condition, including paperwork from your employer, your insurer, and the government. Also, you need to make copies of all documents you submit and correspondence you write to anyone about your condition. You may never need all the paperwork, but it can be essential to your case if you have trouble with a benefits claim.

▮ Understanding Social Security

The Social Security Administration oversees a number of disability programs, including programs that provide monthly cash to people with disabilities. Don't expect a financial windfall; the monthly stipend barely covers the basic expenses. To qualify for programs under Social Security, you must meet certain criteria.

- You cannot hold a job that pays more than $860 a month.
- You can no longer do the work you used to do.
- Your Parkinson's disease prevents you from doing other sedentary work. (Sedentary work requires the ability to lift up to 10 pounds, sit six hours a day, and occasionally walk or stand the remaining two hours of an eight-hour work day.)
- Your disability will last at least a year.

You can get a better idea of your eligibility for assistance by reviewing the Benefit Eligibility Screening Tool (BEST) online at http://best.ssa.gov/. For more information, call Social Security on weekdays at 800-772-1213.

If you qualify, you may be eligible for some of the following programs.

Social Security Disability Insurance

Social Security Disability Insurance (SSDI) covers people younger than age 65 who have worked for pay and are now disabled. The amount of the monthly benefit depends on your income during the working period.

Supplemental Security Income

Supplemental Security Income (SSI) provides monthly cash to people who are disabled and need low-income assistance. This program is based only on financial need; it is typically provided to people with limited work history and to people who are waiting for their SSDI coverage to begin.

To qualify for SSI, a person must have very few assets. For example, under current rules, a single person must have total assets worth less than $2,000 and income under $638 a month, making it difficult for these people to accept part-time work.

■ Health Insurance

As soon as you learn you have PD, you need to begin developing an insurance strategy. I had health insurance through my employer when I was working, but by the time I left that job, I couldn't afford the payments to continue my coverage for the period between leaving my job and qualifying for Medicare coverage.

You need to be familiar with both public health-care plans—Medicare and Medicaid—and various private insurance options. These programs can be quite confusing and the rules change on a regular basis. Following is a brief description of the programs, along with contact information.

Medicare

Medicare is a federal health insurance program for people over the age of 65 and for people with disabilities who can't work. Medicare doesn't cover every medical bill, but it can help. People with Parkinson's who qualify for SSDI automatically qualify for Medicare after being considered disabled and approved for SSDI for 24 months. It makes no sense to me to have to wait for your Medicare benefits, but that's the law. Both Michael and I struggled during this coverage gap with fear that we would not be able to afford our medication and pay for doctor visits when paying our other living expenses.

Medicare is divided into two components:

- ■ *Medicare Part A* helps pay for expenses in hospitals, skilled nursing facilities, hospices (for people who are dying), and nursing homes. It will not pay for daily custodial care.
- ■ *Medicare Part B* covers doctors, diagnostic tests, outpatient hospital services, physical therapy, medical equipment and supplies, and ambulance services. It is available for a monthly fee. To qualify for benefits, your doctor must certify in writing

that you need the care to manage your Parkinson's disease. Keep a copy of this written statement and show it to your pharmacist when you make a purchase. There are many items that Medicare won't cover, so check with the program before making a purchase if you aren't sure whether it will be covered.

■ Recent changes to the law permit coverage of prescription drugs. Plans vary widely; be sure to compare plans before making a selection.

To learn more about Medicare, call 800-633-4227 and ask for a copy of materials related to Parkinson's or visit www.medicare.gov or www.cms.hhs.gov (the websites for the Centers for Medicare and Medicaid Services) to get the information online. For a detailed explanation of Medicare and a free copy of *Your Medicare Handbook,* call the Social Security Administration at 800-772-1213.

Medigap and Medicare HMOs

Private insurance companies sell Medigap insurance to fill in the gap and cover costs not included under Medicare. Medicare HMOs usually replace traditional Medicare policies; they require you to choose from a fixed group of doctors and health-care providers. You cannot be denied Medigap insurance if you apply within six months of first applying for Medicare Part B. You cannot be denied coverage by a Medicare HMO as long as you select the policy during an annual open-enrollment period. Compare policies carefully; coverage can vary dramatically.

You can learn the latest information about Medigap insurance and Medicare HMOs from the booklet *Guide to Health Insurance for People with Medicare,* which is provided by the Social Security Administration and updated every year. (See contact information above.)

Medicaid

Medicaid is a federal and state health-care assistance program for the poor, disabled, senior citizens, and children. States determine eligibility requirements and benefits. Contact your state's Medicaid office for more information.

State Health Insurance Counseling and Assistance Programs

Every state offers SHIP programs to help Medicare recipients find the best insurance options. Information about these state programs is available at http://www.medicare.gov/contacts/static/allStateContacts. asp.

Private Insurance

When it comes to traditional insurance, health insurance companies vary greatly on what costs they will cover. Before you sign up for a health insurance plan, answer the following questions:

- How much is the monthly premium?
- How high is the deductible?
- How much are the copayments?
- Are prescription medications covered?
- Must medication be purchased through a specific pharmacy?
- Is there an exclusion for preexisting conditions? If so, how long do I have to wait before treatment for my Parkinson's disease to be covered? (Typically, the wait is 6 or 12 months.)
- Are there caps to the coverage?
- Does the plan cover the services of specialists, such as neurologists or movement-disorders specialists?

If you're working, you may be eligible to buy health insurance through your employer or through a professional, trade, or religious association. (If an employer offers health insurance to one employee, the same offer must be extended to all employees.) You may need to reveal your Parkinson's status at the time you purchase the insurance. Fees and benefits vary widely from provider to provider; you may be able to get coverage for your children or spouse for an additional fee.

You may also buy an individual health insurance policy. It can be very difficult—and expensive—for someone with Parkinson's disease to qualify for individual health insurance. Worse still, individual plans often charge higher rates for inferior coverage, compared to group plans.

Contact your state insurance commission to find out if the state offers a high-risk health insurance pool, a plan available to people who are denied insurance elsewhere. While these policies can be costly, many states do provide this as an option for people with Parkinson's disease and other chronic conditions.

Consolidated Omnibus Budget Reconciliation Act

The Consolidated Omnibus Budget Reconciliation Act (COBRA) is a federal law requiring your employer to extend coverage under the company's group plan for a fixed amount of time to former employees who assume the cost of the premiums. Any employee can extend COBRA benefits for up to 18 months; someone who qualifies as disabled under the Social Security guidelines can extend that period to 29 months. In most cases, the cost of COBRA insurance is lower than the cost of a short-term health insurance policy. COBRA also applies to the employee's dependents in the event of divorce or death.

Once you have been laid off or quit your job, you have up to 60 days to accept COBRA benefits. Employers with fewer than 20 employees, the federal government, companies that go out of business, and churches are exempt from COBRA, though many still provide COBRA benefits.

Health Insurance Portability and Accountability Act of 1996

This law protects people with Parkinson's disease and other health problems from being discriminated against by insurers and employers. It states that all employees must be offered health insurance at the same price, regardless of their health status. In addition, it forbids insurance companies that offer individual policies from excluding coverage for people with preexisting conditions if they have had continuous coverage in a group plan for the previous 18 months, are not eligible for coverage under a group plan, and have used up their COBRA benefits.

The law also allows you to maintain your health insurance when you change jobs. If you have been diagnosed with Parkinson's disease for more than six months and have had continuous coverage in an insurance plan and then leave your job, you cannot be denied insurance by your new employer because of a preexisting condition. If you have been diagnosed within the six months before you change jobs, your new employer has the right to limit your health insurance for up to one year.

▌ Hiring an Attorney

If you can possibly afford to do so, I highly recommend that you hire an attorney when you apply for Social Security Disability or any other benefits. I waited two years to hire a lawyer, and I didn't get anywhere until I had help. Michael hired an attorney and he received benefits within seven months. The system can be complicated, and it can be beneficial to work with an expert who can help you navigate the bureaucracy. Most Social Security lawyers do not require payment in advance; instead, they are paid when you receive your disability check. I do not recommend hiring an attorney who wants money in advance. Do not be afraid to talk to several attorneys before making a decision about who to hire.

Here are some questions to ask.

I How long have you been working on disability cases?
I How many cases have you won?
I What is your fee for service if I receive disability?
I What experience do you and your firm have handling Social Security?
I If I were to hire you, what would the time line of my case look like? What would you need me to do?

If you do not get satisfactory answers or do not feel comfortable with an attorney for any reason, interview another one. You may also want to contact your local bar association and ask for a listing of attorneys who specialize in disability law.

I Medical Assistance Programs

In some cases, people with Parkinson's can be caught in a period without medical coverage. Since Medicare coverage doesn't become effective until about two years from the time Social Security declares you disabled, some of us are left uninsured for a period of months.

I found myself without any insurance for a while when I moved to Florida. My medications cost more than $1,800 a month, and I simply didn't have the money. I had to discontinue all of the meds except Sinemet because I couldn't afford them. On occasion I would run out of medication three or four days before my next disability check would arrive, and I'd have to stay in bed, unable to function.

I now know about medication assistance programs offered by the pharmaceutical companies that manufacture Parkinson's drugs. Many of these programs provide Parkinson's medications to patients for free or at reduced cost.

▐ Drug Assistance Websites ▐

A number of websites carry useful information for people with Parkinson's disease.

www.disabilityresources.org
www.helpingpatients.org
www.medicare.gov/AssistancePrograms/Home.asp
www.medicationfoundation.com
www.needymeds.com
www.rxassist.org
www.themedicineprogram.com

Additional programs may also be available. I recommend that you search the Internet using the key words "drug assistance" and the name of your state.

▐ Other Government Assistance Programs

Don't be shy about availing yourself of all of the local, state, and federal assistance programs that might be offered in your area. I recommend that you work with a PD advocate in your state who may be more familiar with the programs that are offered. At the risk of sounding melodramatic, for some of us, these programs can sometimes make the difference between eating and not eating.

For many of us, the reality of PD forces us to rethink our financial future and options. We may have to accept more financial assistance than we ever thought we would, but it is essential to remain open-minded about how to handle these issues. In some cases, we have to adjust our financial expectations and lower our standards of living. When I was able to work, I made a good living and saved for what I had always assumed would be a secure and reasonably comfortable retirement decades later. Things didn't turn out that way: My work life ended in my forties, not my sixties or seventies, and I have had to spend the money I once earmarked for my later years.

It hasn't been easy, but I have come to accept these changes, in the same way that I have rethought who I am—and who I will be— in other aspects of my life. Chapter 17 explores some of the many other ways that PD forces people with Parkinson's to discover new things about ourselves. Too often PD is financially devastating, as it was for me, but it can also open us to new possibilities that may never have been available without the experience of surviving with Parkinson's disease.

17

Rediscover Yourself: Redefining What You Have to Offer the World

"I'm a writer and a poet and an advocate, things I never thought I'd be," said Marian, a 60-year-old Chicago woman with Parkinson's disease. "There's an amazing thing that happens to those of us with Parkinson's: one door closes and God opens another. For some odd reason, creativity in one form or another—it could be music or writing or painting or dance or photography—it comes out."

After her diagnosis, Marian began writing poetry; her work was honored at the World Parkinson Congress. "I believe it's all due to the Parkinson's," she said. "I believe that one part of the brain dies off and another part takes over, and for many of us, that new strength is creativity."

Studies have found that Marian is right. Many people with Parkinson's do tap into hidden creative forces that they have either ignored or failed to fully realize before the illness took hold. Many people with Parkinson's discover a new appreciation for language or art—even dance. Ironically, people with Parkinson's who can barely walk across a room can often glide, their movements flowing, when they set their movement to music and dance. How? Researchers suspect that a different part of the brain is used to activate movement associated with dance or other creative activities.

"I've always been a musician," said James, a Texan. "I'm a guitar player, and my first thought when I was diagnosed was that I'm going to lose the music. That was what I was most afraid of. When I play, the Parkinson's goes away. I can tremor and have dyskinesia, but when I start to play, the symptoms fade away. I'm not as good as I used to be, but I can hold my own. And when I'm having a good night, the music flows."

Parkinson's transforms the people it touches. In addition to stimulating creativity, it can also allow us to rediscover our faith, our sense of humor, or our mission as advocates for causes greater than ourselves. This chapter will explore some of the opportunities presented to people with Parkinson's to rediscover themselves and to achieve new goals they may never have imagined in the days before their diagnosis.

"This is not how I envisioned my life," said Sarah, who was diagnosed with PD at age 57. "Once I got through the depression, I realized that the only choice I had was how I was going to handle it. We have every minute of every day to be thankful for. We need to do what we want to do, say what we want to say, and go where we want to go. Parkinson's is not a death sentence. In some ways, it has actually made me more alive."

▌ Remaking Yourself

Parkinson's disease forces you to look closely at who you are and make decisions about what you want to do with your life. You may need to change your career, revise your dreams, and rebuild your relationships, but with change comes opportunity.

Before I developed PD, I defined myself through my career as an educator and my role as a wife and mother. Parkinson's forced me to change careers and to adapt my personal relationships with my family. I am still an educator, but rather than teaching autistic children in a school setting, I teach everyone I can about Parkinson's disease. I am still a mother and partner, but my relationships have changed—in many ways they have become more honest and fulfilling. I do not allow Parkinson's disease to define who I am, but it has helped me to channel my energy into becoming much stronger in many important ways.

We have a chance to remake ourselves every day. Every morning I wake up, God willing. Then I make the decision to get up and put my feet on the floor. Some days I fall flat on my face, but I pick myself up and try again. There are always obstacles to overcome, but the most important determination of how I view my day is my attitude toward those obstacles. There are no rules with this disease; it's up to each of us to do the best we can each day. We won't experience success by ignoring the Parkinson's but by adapting our lives to be successful with Parkinson's.

"I'm Not Sure I Wouldn't Choose to Have This Disease"

Tom, 67, was an orthopedic surgeon before developing Parkinson's disease. This is his story.

I was a surgeon at the time my right hand developed a tremor. I had trouble holding my instrument in the operating room. I had a resting tremor, not an intention tremor, so the tremor stopped as soon as I moved. I thought I had carpal tunnel syndrome, but it was Parkinson's.

Once I was diagnosed, I quit surgery. I went into a tailspin and became depressed and withdrawn. I lost my zip.

With the passage of time, things started to mellow, but I had to go through the grieving process. Over time, I have built my life with its limitations.

I'm not sure I wouldn't choose to have this disease. When you have an irreversible condition and you can no longer do the things you did, there is a vacuum and you find another way to fill it. I'm a painter now. I've deepened my relations with my family and my church. I am deliberate in the things I do.

Before the Parkinson's, I was conditioned to respond. I feel I was in a stadium watching the game, and I had to change my seat. I see life from a completely different angle now. I have a different perspective. I am more tender, a more gentle spirit now. I am more focused and more developed as a person.

I think the most significant change is the realization that life is finite. Time is running out and I'm not the least bit depressed about that. I have no regrets. I plan to end with a sense of promise. I am enjoying the twilight years.

▌ Discover Your Creativity

I don't believe that Parkinson's disease will turn you into a Michelangelo if all you could draw before your diagnosis was stick figures, but I do think that people better utilize their creative skills after they have PD. For some, it may be that they have more time to devote to the discipline required for creative pursuits; others may feel more open and expressive through their art.

You had skills and talents before PD, and you have skills and talents afterward, too. You may have to modify what you do to some degree, but you do not need to close down creatively. I have always enjoyed photography, but I think my eye has improved in the years since I developed PD. I see color differently; I see images in the moment and imagine them as photographs. Once I held a potato chip in one hand and balanced my camera on my knee while a seagull came down to me. I snapped the picture as the bird approached me; I caught every feather while he was in flight. I found it a delightful experience.

I want to paint in bright colors when my meds aren't working. I want to capture the movement of my tremors, both the violence and the flow. I plan to call it "Park Art"—that seems to say it all.

Somehow when we are creative, the Parkinson's symptoms tend to subside. I know people with Parkinson's who sing in barbershop quartets and church choirs; they stammer and whisper in traditional speech, but sing in a loud and pure voice. I sing in my church choir and while I do better on some days than others, the euphoric feeling I have when I'm singing outweighs anything else going on at that time.

I can lose my balance walking across the room, but I can dance without missing a beat. Studies have actually found that people who put on uplifting music and dance experience an improvement in their quality of life, even if they don't experience an improvement in their Parkinson's symptoms when the music is off.

It's up to you to decide how to express yourself and what you want to say, but I challenge you to grant yourself permission to get creative. You will almost certainly find that you have hidden gifts that you may not have been aware of before you developed your PD symptoms.

■ Discover Your Mission

Many people with Parkinson's find empowerment through advocacy, either on behalf of Parkinson's issues or other concerns that they consider important. One of the frustrations of Parkinson's disease is that we lose the power over the movement of our bodies; political advocacy allows us to experience the power of standing up on behalf of a cause greater than ourselves.

"Though this disease, I've learned that I'm good at politics," said James, 51, who has lobbied on behalf of Parkinson's disease issues at both the state and the national level. "For some reason, I'm good at it. I can make a difference and that part makes me feel good. I've gone from being a nine-to-five workaday dad to being a leader. My daughter is proud of me. I suppose I've found a cause—or a cause has found me."

Both Michael and I realized that there was a need to help people with Parkinson's who are essentially alone. We strive to educate people about Parkinson's and to support laws that provide fair opportunities for those of us with the disease.

Frankly, Parkinson's is not a sexy disease. Most people dismiss PD as a disease of the elderly. It's far too easy for lawmakers to treat those of us with Parkinson's as if we are invisible. We want people to become educated and outspoken about the issues that concern them.

Advocacy is therapy. When we work toward helping someone else, we stop focusing on poor, pitiful me and what I need; when we focus on other people, we nurture ourselves. I think that people with Parkinson's need to be their own advocates. If we don't stand up for ourselves, who will do it for us?

Carol, 63, has found strength through her work as a Parkinson's advocate. "When I was first diagnosed, I asked 'Why me?'" she said. "Then a friend said, 'Why not you?' That was all it took for me to see my disease differently. I saw that I needed to make something good come of it." Carol became an advocate with the Parkinson's Action Network and travels to Washington, D.C., once a year to lobby on behalf of issues of concern to people with Parkinson's. "Being part of a bigger group makes me feel like I'm not alone. It gives my connection to the illness a greater meaning."

■ Discover Your Faith

After we learn we have Parkinson's disease, many of us lose faith in God—and others find our faith grows stronger. While we have had times when we've questioned God and been angry at him, both Michael and I have found strength in our faith. I cannot tell you what to believe, but no matter what form your religion or spiritual expression takes, I do believe that a faith in the order of the universe as it makes sense to you will help you make sense of life with Parkinson's disease.

We have received great comfort from our support group at church. We tell others that their place of worship may be a great place to help them start a support group. Our group is not only for those with PD but for those who are affected with a variety of neurological issues, such as multiple sclerosis, muscular dystrophy, stroke, and other problems. It is also not only for the patients, but for their caregivers as well, and for people whose lives have not been touched by illness but who are interested in helping those around them.

I know there is a purpose in this illness for me. I'm certainly not glad that I developed PD, but I consider the people I've met and many of the experiences I've had because of my illness to be among the greatest blessings in my life. I believe that God has a purpose for my life—including my life with PD—and it's up to me to discover that meaning and live it to its fullest. This may not have been the life that I had imagined when I was 25 years old and felt that anything was possible, but this is the life that God has chosen for me.

"Parkinson's has strengthened my faith," said Michael. "I have spent many nights and days looking for direction and hope, and I now see how this disease has drawn me closer to God. Some people question God and lose their faith. They ask God, 'How could you let this happen to me?' What wisdom I have tells me that God didn't cause the Parkinson's, but God can help bring us through."

Of course, it's impossible to give faith to another person, but I do encourage you to reflect on the blessings in your life and to try to determine what your spiritual mission may be. The big questions in life are no different than they were before diagnosis, but when you're living with a debilitating illness, it's much easier to become bitter and lose confidence in the virtue of the world. This disease cannot take away your joy unless you let it. Talk to friends and family, clergy and spiritual advisers, whoever is willing to acknowledge his or her own journey in search of meaning. These discussions can help you focus your thoughts, and they will help you feel closer to your loved ones—and closer to God.

▌ Discover Your Sense of Humor

I believe in the healing power of laughter. At first, all of the harsh realities of living with Parkinson's disease seem completely humorless, but over time you may learn to laugh at yourself and your misfortune. When Michael and I stumble and fall, we check to make sure the fallen is safe and uninjured, then we score the fall on a 10-point scale (based on grace, style, and form).

Laughter is good medicine. A good laugh makes you feel better. It allows you to feel amused rather than embarrassed or ashamed, and it puts others around you at ease. (If she's laughing at herself, they think, she must be doing okay.) We aren't intentionally performing a slapstick routine by falling or flinging our food from our plates, but we might as well see the humor in the moment when it happens. Given the choice between depression and laughter, I go for the laugh every time.

■ Discover New Skills

Parkinson's disease has truly been both a blessing and curse: I feel cursed by the loss of control over the movement of my body, but also blessed with the realization that I am so much more than my physical self. This disease has allowed me to develop new skills that I never imagined I possessed. I have become a national advocate, a political organizer, a Parkinson's educator, a suicide-prevention counselor, a psychotherapist, a true friend—and more. Don't focus your attention on the things you can no longer do; instead, take stock of the many things you can do that you had never dreamed possible.

Actor Michael J. Fox refuses to be defined by his Parkinson's. Instead, he claims it has made him a "fuller person." Says Fox: "I'm living with it. And it is okay. I'm still me—me with Parkinson's."

While I am grateful for all that I have learned about myself as I have lived with Parkinson's, I still long for a cure. Every day I work to support those working toward a cure—and every night I pray that Parkinson's disease will someday become a disease of the past. Chapter 18 explores possible treatments that may someday be the answer to my prayers.

▌ Michael's Fish Story ▌

One of my greatest pleasures is fishing. There is a lake out back where I drop a line each morning in search of freshwater bass. You may be wondering, how can a guy with Parkinson's—whose morning tremors are so bad—go fishing? Aha, I say. That's my secret. The fish like all that shaking. My tremors make those rubber worms dance, and the fish just can't resist the temptation to take a bite.

Yes, there are days when my meds are off and the tremors are out of control, making fishing an exercise in futility. I've been stabbed with hooks, dropped my pole in the water, and gotten tangled in the fishing line. I consider these my therapy days, the days that test my ability to persevere in the face of adversity. It's not about whether I catch any fish; it's about my personal challenge to overcome the Parkinson's symptoms and continue fishing. I'm sure my neighbors look out their windows and take pity on the poor shaking man at the lake. I don't care what they think. This is my race, my challenge, my test—and I'm going fishing.

18

Hope: New Horizons in Parkinson's Disease Treatments

Every day of my life I pray for a cure for Parkinson's disease. Hope is essential, and I am genuinely optimistic that a cure will be discovered in my lifetime.

While researchers are exploring new medications and approaches to surgery to control the symptoms of Parkinson's, I believe the future of a cure will most likely involve gene therapy or stem-cell transplants. This chapter will review some of the ongoing research and new approaches to treating Parkinson's disease that are currently in development.

▌A Note from Michael's Son ▌

During the time Michael and I have been working on this book, his entire family has been swept up in the need to communicate about Parkinson's. Michael's young son has become his own Parkinson's advocate. Here's what he wrote.

My name is Michael J. Church Jr., and I want to tell you about Parkinson's disease because my dad has it. Ever since I was a little kid, my dad has had Parkinson's. I feel really bad half of the time. Every day his Parkinson's gets worse and worse. Most of the time I would rather have it instead of him having it.

We need to find a cure. I miss things that I used to do with my dad, like camping and playing around more than he can now. The faster we can find a cure, the more stuff my dad can do. I do not like to see him sick. I also do not like it that other people with Parkinson's have to suffer. It would be good to have my dad better. I bet there are other kids who have parents with Parkinson's who want their moms and dads better, too.

▌ Gene Therapy

Gene therapy involves using a harmless virus to introduce a gene into another cell. In the case of Parkinson's disease, the gene is introduced into a part of the brain known as the subthalamic nucleus, where it stimulates the production of the neurotransmitter GABA.

For more than five years, researchers have experimented with gene therapy to control Parkinson's symptoms in rats and monkeys with Parkinson-like symptoms. The results have been promising: Studies have shown significant ongoing clinical benefit, and the procedure appears safe, even after five years of follow-up.

Early research shows the approach works on humans, too. The first human clinical trial of gene therapy treatment for Parkinson's disease suggests that the approach can significantly reduce PD symptoms. According to a report issued in October 2006, a one-year trial including 12 people with Parkinson's showed an average of 25 percent improvement in motor control. (Nine of the participants showed an average improvement of 37 percent, and one had a 65 percent improvement, based on the unified Parkinson's disease rating scale.)

In addition, none of the participants showed signs of reduced immunity, one of the serious complications of gene therapy that has caused problems in trials for other illnesses. The researchers plan long-term monitoring of the study participants to look for immune system problems or other side effects.

As part of the treatment, researchers engineered a harmless virus designed to carry genes that are encoded with a protein called glutamic acid decarboxylase, or GAD. (Viruses are very effective at inserting their genetic material into cells.) The protein helps make a key nerve-signaling chemical called gamma aminobutyric acid (GABA), which inhibits a region of the brain that is overactive in people with Parkinson's. The virus is introduced by injecting a tiny drop of a solution containing the virus directly into the brain. The study participants were undergoing deep brain stimulation surgery at the time the treatment was administered; the efficacy of the gene therapy was assessed when the DBS device was turned off.

While the results were quite dramatic, researchers theorize that treating a larger area of the subthalamic nucleus of the brain could yield even more impressive results. The U.S. Food and Drug Administration has approved a gene therapy clinical trial at the University of California at San Francisco designed to determine the safety and efficacy of gene therapy when administered at several different dosages.

Another approach still in development involves using a catheter to infuse GDNF—glial-derived neurotrophic factor—into the basal ganglia in the brain. In the body, the GDNF triggers the formation of levodopa. This technique is not yet available, even for animal research.

▌ Stem-Cell Therapy

There has been a lot of debate about the use of stem cells, particularly when it comes to embryonic stem cells. There has also been a lot of misinformation about the issue. Currently the research being done on adult stem cells uses cord-blood stem cells, and it is showing promise in the treatment of several diseases. However, adult stem cells have yet to be found to adapt and become any type of cell in the body. For those with PD and other neurological issues, adult stem cells have yet to be able to become the needed nerve and brain cells that will help our situation.

Parkinson's disease may be one of the first illnesses that can be treated using stem-cell transplantation because researchers know the specific type of cells—DA neurons—needed to relieve the symptoms. In addition, researchers have been able to induce embryonic stem cells to develop into DA neurons in a laboratory.

Researchers have transplanted mouse embryonic stem cells that were differentiated into DA neurons into the brains of rats with Parkinson's symptoms. The experiment was a success. The rats treated with the stem cells generated new neurons that were able to release dopamine and reverse the Parkinsonian symptoms.

Will the same approach work in humans? Many researchers believe it will. Currently scientists are working on generating human stem cells differentiated into DA neurons that could be transplanted into the human brain. While federal funding for the research remains in the hands of the politicians at this point, many researchers believe that human stem-cell transplantation will be available in the future.

▌ New Drugs to Treat Parkinson's Symptoms

Researchers are attempting to develop new drugs to treat Parkinson's symptoms that are more effective and have fewer side effects than levodopa. Drugs in development include:

▌ *New dopamine agonists.* These drugs, including sumanirole, which is currently in drug trials, would last longer than existing dopamine agonists, minimizing wear-off and possibly lower the risk of dyskinesia.

▌ *Dopamine patch.* Providing drugs through a 24-hour transdermal patch would allow a more steady delivery of medication, possibly minimizing off time.

▌ *Drugs to minimize dyskinesia.* Medications known as alpha–2-adrenoreceptor antagonists and 5-HT1A agonists may reduce the risk of dyskinesia associated with the use of levodopa. Animal studies have found the drug effective at dramatically reducing dyskinesia, one of the most debilitating side effects of levodopa.

▌ *Neuroprotective drugs.* These medications are designed to protect the dopamine-producing cells in the brain. Theoretically, these drugs could slow the progress of the disease to the point that a person could have decades of motor function control before the symptoms became serious enough to require additional treatment. Some researchers are optimistic about the development of such a drug in the next decade or so.

▌ *Neurotrophic agents.* Neurotrophic agents help to repair damaged brain cells and encourage the growth of new cells. Researchers have studied GDNF in animal studies involving Parkinson's disease and found the agent assisted in the regeneration of damaged dopamine-producing brain cells. Human studies in which the GDNF was delivered into the spinal fluid of the brain were not successful; current research focuses on delivering the GDNF directly to the brain cells that need it. In addition, researchers are exploring other neurotrophic growth factors, including fibroblast growth factor (FGF), ciliary neurotrophic factor (CNTF), and brain-derived neurotrophic factor (BDNF), among others.

▌ *GM1 ganglioside.* GM1 ganglioside (GM1) is a chemical in the cell membrane that helps injured dopamine cells to recover. Animal studies involving monkeys have shown that the monkeys' motor symptoms significantly decreased after treatment with GM1 for six to eight weeks. A 16-week human study involving 45 people with Parkinson's found significant improvement in rigidity and bradykinesia in the group treated with GM1. Additional research is ongoing.

▌ Our Hope

Clearly, there is reason to be optimistic about future treatments for Parkinson's disease. Researchers are making headway toward the development of new drugs that may improve symptoms with minimal side effects as well as procedures that may be able to restore the dopamine-producing cells in the brain, effectively curing the disease.

While we wait for these safer and more effective treatments to be tested and approved, each of us with Parkinson's disease can take the steps necessary to live well in the moment. Marian, 60, isn't waiting for a cure. "I don't think Parkinson's disease will be cured in my lifetime," she said, "but that's okay. I try to teach people how to live well with the disease. I think that's more important. It's all we can really do for ourselves."

You must accept the reality that you have Parkinson's disease—and then you must overcome it by not allowing your physical limitations to define your way of life. Focus on your strengths and your abilities: remember what you can do, instead of dwelling on the things you may no longer be able to do.

Our hope is that, after reading this book, you no longer feel alone. Others with the disease are finding ways to achieve their dreams. The diagnosis of Parkinson's disease is not a death sentence; you can live a long, productive, and joyful life. I encourage you to appreciate the many blessings of your life with Parkinson's so that you can live well with the disease while we are waiting together for the research that will bring us all one step closer to a cure.

APPENDIX

Medication Charts

I am forever tinkering with the medicines I take, and I could never remember the specifics if I didn't write them down. Here are two formats that you might find useful in recording your information and sharing it with your doctor. Feel free to copy these charts and take them with you to your doctor's appointments.

Whatever format you use, be sure to keep detailed notes, especially in the beginning. Take note of your daily stress, exercise patterns, and any other information you think might be useful. If necessary, note whether or not you're having trouble sleeping or if you begin to feel depressed or lonely. Think of these charts as data, measurements of how your condition is changing and responding to treatment. By having this information available, your doctor can assess your progress, even if you are having an abnormally on or off day during your visit.

Medication History

Date	Time	Dosage	Symptoms/Mood	Stress/Activity
____	____	____	_____	_____
____	____	____	_____	_____
____	____	____	_____	_____

24-Hour Record of Symptoms

Date: _____

Time	Medication Dosage	Symptoms/Mood/Stress/Activity
6 A.M.	_____	_____
8 A.M.	_____	_____
10 A.M.	_____	_____
12 P.M.	_____	_____
2 P.M.	_____	_____
4 P.M.	_____	_____
6 P.M.	_____	_____
8 P.M.	_____	_____
10 P.M.	_____	_____
12 A.M.	_____	_____
2 A.M.	_____	_____
4 A.M.	_____	_____

RESOURCES

■ Organizations of Interest

American Parkinson Disease Association
1250 Hylan Blvd., Suite 4B
Staten Island, NY 10305
(800) 223-2732; (718) 981-8001
www.apdaparkinson.com
Provides education, patient and family support, and research on Parkinson's disease; offers a newsletter and a resource guide.

Caregiver Media Group
3005 Greene St.
Hollywood, FL 33020
(800) 829-2734; (954) 893-0550
www.caregiver.com
Provides information and support for caregivers of the chronically ill.

Coalition for the Advancement of Medical Research
2021 K St. NW, Suite 305
Washington, DC 20006

(202) 293-2856
www.camradvocacy.org
Dedicated to advancing stem-cell research.

Grassroots Connection
www.grassrootsconnection.com
Provides online information and advocacy opportunities for people interested in supporting laws beneficial to people with Parkinson's and other neurological diseases.

Michael J. Fox Foundation for Parkinson's Research
Grand Central Station
PO Box 4777
New York, NY 10163
(800) 708-7644
www.michaeljfox.org
Raises money to support research on finding a cure for Parkinson's disease.

Motivating Moves
1359 Broadway, Suite 1509
New York, NY 10018
(800) 457-6676
www.motivatingmoves.com
Sells a DVD and video of a seated exercise program for people with Parkinson's disease; cost: $14.95. (This program is sponsored by the Parkinson's Disease Foundation.)

Movers & Shakers
15275 Collier Blvd., #201
Box 151
Naples, FL 34119
(239) 431-6139

www.pdoutreach.org
   Provides support and advocacy for people with young-onset Parkinson's disease.

National Family Caregivers Association
10400 Connecticut Ave., Suite 500
Kensington, MD 20895
(800) 896-3650; (301) 942-6430
www.nfcacares.org
   Provides support to caregivers of the chronically ill.

National Institute of Neurological Disorders and Stroke
NIH Neurological Institute
PO Box 5801
Bethesda, MD 20824
(800) 352-9424
www.ninds.nih.gov
   This division of the National Institutes of Health supports and conducts research on the nervous system, including Parkinson's disease.

National Parkinson Foundation, Inc.
Bob Hope Parkinson Research Center
1501 NW Ninth Ave.
Miami, FL 33136-1494
(800) 327-4545; (305) 547-6666
www.parkinson.org
   Resource for general information, publications, and news reports; publishes The Parkinson Report, *a quarterly journal.*

Parkinson's Action Network
1025 Vermont Ave. NW, Suite 1120
Washington, DC 20005

(800) 850-4726; (202) 638-4101
www.parkinsonsaction.org
 Promotes research and advocacy regarding issues of concern to people with Parkinson's disease.

The Parkinson Alliance
211 College Road E, 3rd Floor
Princeton, NJ 08520
(800) 579-8440; (609) 688-0870
www.parkinsonalliance.net
 Raises money to support research on Parkinson's disease.

Parkinson's Disease Foundation
1359 Broadway, Suite 1509
New York, NY 10018
(800) 457-6676; (212) 923-4700
www.pdf.org
 Supports worldwide research into the causes and cure of Parkinson's disease through the use of internationally supported grant programs; publishes the quarterly journals PDF News *and the* PDF Science Bulletin.

The Parkinson's Institute
1170 Morse Ave.
Sunnyvale, CA 94089-1605
(408) 734-2800; (800) 786-2958
www.parkinsonsinstitute.org
 Seeks a cure for Parkinson's disease and other movement disorders; also explores more effective diagnostic and treatment methods.

Parkinson's Resource Organization
74090 El Paseo, Suite 102

Palm Desert, CA 92260-4135
(877) 775-4111; (760) 773-5628
www.parkinsonsresource.org
   *Strives to educate and emotionally support the families
of people with Parkinson's disease; raises money to support
respite care for caregivers.*

Parkinson's Training for Caregivers

c/o Northwest Parkinson's Foundation
PO Box 56
Mercer Island, WA 98040
(877) 980-7500
www.parkinsonseducator.com
   *Provides a free online course to train caregivers of Parkin-
son's patients; the site is supported by the U.S. Department
of Health and Human Services.*

We Move

204 W 84th St.
New York, NY 10024
www.wemove.org
   *Provides education about the treatment and management
of Parkinson's disease and other neurological movement
disorders.*

World Parkinson Congress

710 W 168th St., 3rd Floor
New York, NY 10032
(800) 457-6676
www.worldpdcongress.org
   *Provides an international forum for scientific discoveries
and medical practices related to Parkinson's disease.*

Young Onset Parkinson's Association
22136 Westheimer Pkwy, Suite 343
Katy, TX 77450
(888) 937-9672
www.yopa.org
    Offers support and advocates on behalf of people with young-onset Parkinson's disease.

■ Websites Offering Information on Clinical Trials

Advancing Parkinson's Therapies: www.pdtrials.org
National Institutes of Health: www.clinicaltrials.gov
Parkinson Pipeline Project: www.pdpipeline.org
Parkinson Study Group: www.parkinson-study-group.org

Online Support Groups
Movers & Shakers: www.pdoutreach.org
Parkinson's Information Exchange Network Online:
www.parkinsons-information-exchange-network-online.com
Parkinson's Partners: http://groups.msn.com/ParkinsonsPartners

Regional and Local Support Groups
Northeast Parkinson's & Caregivers, Inc.:
www.northeastparkinsons.com
Northwest Parkinson's Foundation:
www.nwpf.org
Parkinson Association of the Carolinas:
www.parkinsonassociation.org
Parkinson's Association of Southwest Florida: www.pasfl.org

CHAPTER NOTES

1 What Is Parkinson's Disease?

Goetz, C. G. 2006. "What's New? Clinical Progression and Staging of Parkinson's Disease." *Journal of Neural Transmission* Suppl. 70:305–308.

Korczyn, A. D., and H. Reichmann. 2006. "Dementia with Lewy Bodies." *Journal of Neurological Science* 248(1-2): 3–8.

Shulman, L. M., et al. 2006. "Subjective Report Versus Objective Measurement of Activities of Daily Living in Parkinson's Disease." *Movement Disorders* 21(6): 794–799.

2 Who Gets Parkinson's Disease?

Chade, A. R., et al. 2006. "Nongenetic Causes of Parkinson's Disease." *Journal of Neural Transmission* Suppl. (70):147–151.

Columbia University College of Physicians and Surgeons, Complete Home Medical Guide. New York: Crown Publishers, 1995, p. 146.

Garwood, E. R., et al. 2006. "Amphetamine Exposure Is Elevated in Parkinson's Disease." *Neurotoxicology* 27(6): 1003–1007.

Marsh, G. M., and M. J. Gula. 2006. "Employment as a

Welder and Parkinson's Disease Among Heavy Equipment Manufacturing Workers." *Journal of Occupational and Environmental Medicine* 48(10): 1031–1046.

Mizuno, Y., et al. 2006. "Progress in Familial Parkinson's Disease." *Journal of Neural Transmission,* Suppl. 70:191–204.

Riess, O., et al. 2006. "Genetic Causes of Parkinson's Disease: Extending the Pathway." *Journal of Neural Transmission,* Suppl. 70:181–189.

3 Do You Have Parkinson's Disease?

Iansek, R., et al. 2006. "The Sequence Effect and Gait Festination in Parkinson's Disease: Contributors to Freezing of Gait? *Movement Disorders* 21(9): 1419–1424.

Katzenschlager, R., and A. J. Lees. 2002. "Treatment of Parkinson's Disease: Levodopa as the First Choice." *Journal of Neurology* 249(Suppl. 2): 1119–1124.

Muller, T., and H. Russ. 2006. "Levodopa, Motor Fluctuations and Dyskinesia in Parkinson's Disease." *Expert Opinions on Pharmacotherapy* 7(13): 1715–1730.

Savitt, J. M., et al. 2006. "Diagnosis and Treatment of Parkinson's Disease." *Journal of Clinical Investigation* 116(7): 1744–1754.

4 Drugs for Parkinson's Disease

Grandas, F., et al. 1998. "Quality of Life in Patients with Parkinson's Disease Who Transfer from Standard Levodopa to Sinemet CR: The Star Study." *Journal of Neurology* 245 (Suppl. 1): S31–S33.

Knoll, J. 1986. "Role of B-Type Monoamine Oxidase Inhibition in the Treatment of Parkinson's Disease: An Update." In *Move-*

ment Disorders, N. S. Shah, ed. New York: Plenum, 1986, pp. 53–81.

Parkinson Study Group. 2000. "Pramipexole vs. Levodopa as Initial Treatment for Parkinson's Disease: A Randomized Controlled Trial." *Journal of the American Medical Association* 284(15): 1931–1938.

Shoulson, I., et al. 1989. (Parkinson Study Group) "Effect of Deprenyl on the Progression of Disability in Early Parkinson's Disease." *New England Journal of Medicine* 321(20): 1364–1371.

5 Surgery for Parkinson's Disease

Diamond, A., and J. Jankovic. 2005. "The Effect of Deep Brain Stimulation on Quality of Life in Movement Disorders." *Journal of Neurology, Neurosurgery, and Psychiatry* 76(9): 1188–1193.

Hamani, C., et al. 2006. "Deep Brain Stimulation for the Treatment of Parkinson's Disease." *Journal of Neural Transmission,* Suppl. 70:393–399.

Houeto, J. L., et al. 2006. "Subthalamic Stimulation in Parkinson's Disease: Behavior and Social Adaptation." *Archives of Neurology* 63(8): 1090–1095.

6 Finding the Right Doctor

Mayor, S. 2006. "Only Specialists Should Diagnose Parkinson's Disease." *British Medical Journal* 333(7557): 14.

Moore, A. 2006. "Parkinson's Disease: Critical Diagnosis." *Health Service Journal* Suppl. 116(6016): 1–4.

7 Exercise: The Importance of Movement

Batile, J., et al. 2000. "Effect of Exercise on Perceived Quality of Life of Individuals with Parkinson's Disease." *Journal of Rehabilitation Research and Development* 37(5): 529–534.

Bergen, J. L., et al. 2002. "Aerobic Exercise Intervention Improves Aerobic Capacity and Movement Initiation in Parkinson's Disease Patients." *NeuroRehabilitation* 17(2): 161–168.

Pacchetti, C., et al. 2000. "Active Music Therapy in Parkinson's Disease: An Integrative Method for Motor and Emotional Rehabilitation." *Psychosomatic Medicine* 62(3): 386–393.

Rodrigues de Paula, F., et al. 2006. "Impact of an Exercise Program on Physical, Emotional, and Social Aspect of Quality of Life of Individuals With Parkinson's Disease." *Movement Disorders* 21(8): 1073–1077.

Scandalis, T. A., et al. 2001. "Resistance Training and Gait Function in Patients with Parkinson's Disease." *American Journal of Physical Medicine and Rehabilitation* 80(1): 38–43.

8 Nourish Yourself: The Importance of Diet and Nutritional Supplements

Chiueh, C. C., et al. 2000. "Neuroprotective Strategies in Parkinson's Disease: Protection Against Progressive Nigral Damage Induced by Free Radicals." *Neurotox Res* 2(2-3): 293–310.

Etminan, M., et al. 2005. "Intake of Vitamin E, Vitamin C, and Carotenoids and the Risk of Parkinson's Disease: A Meta-analysis." *Lancet Neurology* 4(6): 362–365.

Jenner, P., and C. W. Olanow. 1996. "Oxidative Stress and the Pathogenesis of Parkinson's Disease." *Neurology* 47(6 Suppl. 3): S161–S170.

Morens, D. M., et al. 1996. "Case-Control Study of Idiopathic

Parkinson's Disease and Dietary Vitamin E Intake." *Neurology* 46(5): 1270–1274.

Sudha, K., et al. 2003. "Free Radical Toxicity and Antioxidants in Parkinson's Disease." *Neurology India* 51(1): 60–62.

Zhang, S. M., et al. 2002. "Intakes of Vitamins E and C, Carotenoids, Vitamin Supplements, and PD Risk." *Neurology* 59(8): 1161–1169.

9 Imagine: The Importance of Attitude and the Mind-Body Connection

Chatterjee, A., et al. 2006. "Art Produced by a Patient with Parkinson's Disease." *Behavioral Neurology* 17(2): 105–108.

Eng, M. L., et al. 2006. "Open-Label Trial Regarding the Use of Acupuncture and Yin Tui na in Parkinson's Disease Outpatients: A Pilot Study on Efficacy, Tolerability, and Quality of Life." *Journal of Alternative and Complementary Medicine* 12(4): 395–399.

Ferry, P., et al. 2002. "Use of Complementary Therapies and Non-prescribed Medication in Patients with Parkinson's Disease." *Postgraduate Medical Journal* 78(924): 612–614.

Paterson, C., et al. 2005. "A Pilot Study of Therapeutic Massage for People with Parkinson's Disease: The Added Value of User Involvement." *Complementary Therapies in Clinical Practice* 11(3): 161–171.

Rajendran, P. R., et al. 2001. "The Use of Alternative Therapies by Patients with Parkinson's Disease." *Neurology* 57(5): 790–794.

Schrag, A., et al. 2001. "Poetic Talent Unmasked by Treatment of Parkinson's Disease." *Movement Disorders* 16(6):1175–1176.

Smith, A. D., et al. 2002. "Stress-Induced Parkinson's Disease: A Working Hypothesis." *Physiology and Behavior* 77(4-5): 527–531.

10 Replenish Yourself: The Importance of Rest and Relaxation

Arnulf, I. 2005. "Excessive Daytime Sleepiness in Parkinsonism." *Sleep Medicine Reviews* 9(3): 185–200.

Comella, C. 2006. "Sleep Disturbances and Excessive Daytime Sleepiness in Parkinson's Disease: An Overview." *Journal of Neural Transmission* Suppl. 70:349–355.

Dowling, G. A., et al. 2005. "Melatonin for Sleep Disturbances in Parkinson's Disease." *Sleep Medicine* 6(5): 459–466.

Gjestad, M. D., et al. 2006. "Excessive Daytime Sleepiness in Parkinson's Disease: Is It the Drugs or the Disease?" *Neurology* 67(5): 853–858.

Lyons, K. E., and R. Pahwa. 2006. "Effects of Bilateral Subthalamic Nucleus Stimulation on Sleep, Daytime Sleepiness, and Early Morning Dystonia in Patients with Parkinson's Disease." *Journal of Neurology* 104(4): 502–505.

Postuma, R. B., et al. 2006. "Potential Early Markers of Parkinson's Disease in Idiopathic REM Sleep Behavior Disorder." *Neurology* 66(6): 845–851.

11 Experience Joy: The Importance of Treating Depression

Borek, L. L., et al. 2006. "Mood and Sleep in Parkinson's Disease." *Journal of Clinical Psychiatry* 67(6): 958–963.

Chung, T. H., et al. 2003. "Systematic Review of Antidepressant Therapies in Parkinson's Disease." *Parkinsonism Related Disorders* 10(2): 59–65.

Kirsch-Darrow, L., et al. 2006. "Dissociating Apathy and Depression in Parkinson's Disease." *Neurology* 67(1): 33–38.

Okun, M. S., and R. L. Watts. 2002. "Depression Associated with Parkinson's Disease: Clinical Features and Treatment." *Neurology* 58(Suppl. 1): S63–S70.

12 Talk: The Importance of Support Groups

Charlton, G. S., and C. J. Barrow. 2002. "Coping and Self-Help Group Membership in Parkinson's Disease: An Exploratory Qualitative Study." *Health and Social Care in the Community* 10(6): 472–478.

Lieberman, M. A., et al. 2005. "Online Support Groups for Parkinson's Patients: A Pilot Study of Effectiveness." *Social Work Health Care* 42(2): 23–38.

Schrag, A., et al. 2000. "How Does Parkinson's Disease Affect Quality of Life? A Comparison with Quality of Life in the General Population." *Movement Disorders* 15(6): 1112–1118.

13 Taking a Break: The Importance of Caring for Your Caregivers

Haberman, B., and L. Davis. 2006. "Lessons Learned from a Parkinson's Disease Caregiver Intervention Pilot Study." *Applied Nursing Research* 19(4): 212–215.

Schrag, A., et al. 2006. "Caregiver Burden in Parkinson's Disease Is Closely Associated with Psychiatric Symptoms, Falls, Disability." *Parkinsonism Related Disorders* 12(1): 35–41.

14 Practical Suggestions for Facing Daily Challenges

Bhatia, S., and A. Gupta. 2003. "Impairments in Activities of Daily Living in Parkinson's Disease: Implications for Management." *NeuroRehabilitation* 18(3): 209–214.

Brichetto, G., et al. 2006. "Evaluation of Physical Therapy in Parkinsonian Patients with Freezing of Gait: A Pilot Study." *Clinical Rehabilitation* 20(1):31–35.

Morris, M. E. 2006. "Locomotor Training in People with Parkinson's Disease." *Physical Therapy* 86(10): 1426–1435.

Thomure, A. 2006. "Helping Your Patient Manage Parkinson's Disease." *Nursing* 36(8): 20–21.

15 Parkinson's Disease Touches Everyone: Working Through Changes in Your Relationships

Calne, S. M. 2003. "The Psychosocial Impact of Late-Stage Parkinson's Disease." *Journal of Neuroscience Nursing* 35(6): 306–313.

Carter, J. H., et al. 1998. "Living with a Person Who Has Parkinson's Disease: The Spouse's Perspective by Stage of Disease: Parkinson's Study Group." *Movement Disorders* 13(1): 20–28.

Greene, S. M., and W. A. Griffin. 1998. "Symptom Study in Context; Effects of Marital Quality on Signs of Parkinson's Disease During Patient-Spouse Interaction." *Psychiatry* 61(1): 35–45.

Schrag, A., et al. 2003. "Young- Versus Older-Onset Parkinson's Disease: Impact of Disease and Psychosocial Consequences." *Movement Disorders* 18(11): 1250–1256.

16 Financial Challenges: Facing Job Loss, Disability, Social Security, and Insurance Struggles

Banks, P., and M. Lawrence. 2006. "The Disability Discrimination Act, A Necessary, But Not Sufficient Safeguard for People with Progressive Conditions in the Workplace? The Experiences of Younger People with Parkinson's Disease." *Disability and Rehabilitation* 28(1): 13–24.

Scheife, R. T., et al. 2000. "Impact of Parkinson's Disease and Its Pharmacologic Treatment on Quality of Life and Economic Outcomes." *American Journal of Health-System Pharmacy* 57(10): 953–962.

17 Rediscover Yourself: Redefining What You Have to Offer the World

Chatterjee, A., et al. 2006. "Art Produced by a Patient with Parkinson's Disease." *Behavioral Neurology* 17(2): 105–108.

Schrag, A., and M. Trimble. 2001. "Poetic Talent Unmasked by Treatment of Parkinson's Disease." *Movement Disorders* 16(6): 1175–1176.

Walker, R. H. 2006. "Augmentation of Artistic Productivity in Parkinson's Disease." *Movement Disorders* 21(2): 285–286.

18 Hope: New Horizons in Parkinson's Disease Treatments

Freed, C. R., et al. 2001. "Transplantation of Embryonic Dopamine Neurons for Severe Parkinson's Disease." *New England Journal of Medicine* 344:710–719.

Khamsi, R. 2006. "Gene Therapy Reduces Parkinson's Symptoms." NewScientist.com, Oct 17, 2006, http://www.newscientist.com/article/dn10317-gene-therapy-reduces-parkinsons-symptoms.html.

Kim J. H., et al. 2002. "Dopamine Neurons Derived from Embryonic Stem Cells Function in an Animal Model of Parkinson's Disease." *Nature* 418:50–56.

Langston, W. 2005. "The Promise of Stem Cells in Parkinson's Disease." *Journal of Clinical Investigation* 115:23–25.

Pope-Coleman, A., and J. S. Schneider. 1998. "Effects of Chronic

GM1 Ganglioside Treatment on Cognitive and Motor Deficits in a Slowly Progressing Model of Parkinsonism in Non-Human Primates." *Restorative Neurology and Neuroscience* 12(4): 255–266.

Pope-Coleman, A., et al. 2000. "Effects of GM1 Ganglioside Treatment on Pre- and Postsynaptic Dopaminergic Markers in the Striatum of Parkinsonian Monkeys." *Synapse* 36(2): 120–128.

INDEX

MRI. *See* Magnetic resonance imaging
Muhammad Ali Parkinson Center, 11
Multiple sclerosis, 144
Multiple systems atrophy, 10
Muscles, strength of, 95
Music, 117
Myobloc (botulinum toxin), 60–61

Naps, 129
National Board of Medical Examiners, 81
National Certification Board for Therapeutic Massage and Bodywork, 119
National Family Caregivers Association, 221
National Institute of Neurological Disorders and Stroke, 221
National Parkinson Foundation, Inc., 221
Neurology, 126, 136
Neuroprotective drugs, 214
Neuro Rehabilitation, 93
Nicotine, 28–29
Numbness, 40
Nutrition, 29, 100–110
  eating well, 107–109
  practical suggestions for facing daily challenges, 162–163
  spicy foods, 108

use of supplements, 100–110
Olfactory changes, 40
Overeating, 129
Oxidative stress, 13

Pallidotomy, 72–74
Paper mills, 25
Parcopa, 57–59
Parents, relationships with, 180–181
Parkinson, James, 11
The Parkinson Alliance, 222
Parkinson's Action Network, 221–222
Parkinson's Disease Foundation, 222
Parkinson's disease (PD), xiii
  age and, 21
  alternative medicine and self-care, xv
  attitude and, 111–123
  caffeine and, 28
  caregivers for, 149–158
  causes of, 11–15
    excitotoxicity, 14
    presence of Lewy bodies, 14–15
    role of mitochondria, 13–14
    role of oxidative stress, 12–13
  changes in relationships and, 171–186
  creativity and, 203–205
  demographics of, 11

ABOUT THE AUTHORS

GRETCHEN GARIE was diagnosed with Parkinson's Disease at age 33. Prior to diagnosis, she worked as an educator specializing in autism and as an autism advocate.

MICHAEL J. CHURCH was diagnosed with Parkinson's Disease at age 32. Before diagnosis, he worked as a mechanic, manager, insurance executive, legislative aide, and political campaign consultant.

Gretchen and Michael are cofounders of Movers & Shakers, a national organization dedicated to providing education and support to others with young-onset Parkinson's Disease. They are also Florida Coordinators for the Parkinson's Action Network. They jointly received the Award of Excellence in Advocacy from the Parkinson's Action Network. In March 2007, Gretchen and Michael married. They live in Naples, Florida.

WINIFRED CONKLING has written more than thirty books on health and medical topics. She lives in Virginia with her husband and three children.